H Forever EALTHY

HFOREVER EALTHY

A Program for a Longer, Better, and Healthier Life

Anthony J. Alosi, MD

iUniverse, Inc.
Bloomington

Forever Healthy
A Program for a Longer, Better, and Healthier Life

The information, ideas, and suggestions in this book are not intended as a substitute for professional medical advice. Before following any suggestions contained in this book, you should consult your personal physician. Neither the author nor the publisher shall be liable or responsible for any loss or damage allegedly arising as a consequence of your use or application of any information or suggestions in this book.

iUniverse books may be ordered through booksellers or by contacting:

iUniverse
1663 Liberty Drive
Bloomington, IN 47403
www.iuniverse.com
1-800-Authors (1-800-288-4677)

Because of the dynamic nature of the Internet, any web addresses or links contained in this book may have changed since publication and may no longer be valid. The views expressed in this work are solely those of the author and do not necessarily reflect the views of the publisher, and the publisher hereby disclaims any responsibility for them.

Any people depicted in stock imagery provided by Thinkstock are models, and such images are being used for illustrative purposes only.
Certain stock imagery © Thinkstock.

ISBN: 978-1-4620-4278-4 (sc)
ISBN: 978-1-4620-4277-7 (hc)
ISBN: 978-1-4620-4354-5 (ebk)

Printed in the United States of America

iUniverse rev. date: 10/15/2011

This book is dedicated to my wife, Virginia Alosi, and my stepdaughter, Mary Rose McNamara, with the help and assistance of David Silver.

CONTENTS

Credits to Jeremy Geffen M.D. For his creation of the
7 Level Program for Healing the Whole Body.

INTRODUCTION

I spent a great deal of my life working with hypnosis. In 1968, I went to the University of Pennsylvania and spent six months working with patients and studying hypnosis. Then, I joined the American Society of Clinical Hypnosis and attended many demonstrations by the great Dr. Milton Erickson. I worked my way up and became certified as a consultant in clinical hypnosis. Since retiring to Florida, I have continued counseling people with problems with anxiety, insomnia, and pain through the use of hypnosis and have recently become a Lifetime Member of the Florida Society of Clinical Hypnosis.

Hypnosis can be considered an alternative medical treatment. Conventional medical practitioners often ignore hypnosis, supplements, and stress treatment in dealing with heart disease, Alzheimer's disease, and other illnesses.

Dr. Stephen T. Sinatra, an integrative cardiologist, has taught that we can prevent and treat heart disease by taking the triad coenzyme Q10 (CoQ10), L-Carnitine, and D-Ribose.

Dr. Dharma Singh Khalsa, in his book *Brain Longevity*, states that chronic stress and cortisol are possible causes of Alzheimer's disease.

I am very unhappy with conventional medicine. Practitioners do blood tests and look for diseases, and then they treat them with toxic drugs. They are only concerned with disease-disease-disease. Thousands of people die every year from prescription drugs.

The future of medicine is anti-aging medicine and bio-identical hormone replacement therapy. I became interested in anti-aging medicine because of Dr. Philip Lee Miller and his book, *Life Extension Revolution*, also Ron Rothenberger's book, *Forever Ageless*. Let us not forget *Ageless* by Suzanne Sommers, in which she interviewed many doctors.

Every morning I apply a transdermal dose of bio-identical testosterone to my inner thighs (100 mg). Then I do the cranial electrotherapy stimulation (CES) of my brain. I attach electrodes with the pads to each ear and send 9 volts of electricity to my brain for twenty minutes. This produces profound relaxation and alpha brain wave stimulation; then I do mindfulness meditation as developed by Dr. Jon Kabot Zinn. This meditation technique makes me a silent witness to my thoughts and the space between my thoughts.

Consistent, concentrated focus helps you to model successful people. I model these five successful individuals: Warren Buffet, Dr. Boercke, Dr. Milton Erickson, Dr. Candice Pert, and Dr. Bruce Lipton.

I model Warren Buffet for stock investments. As a medical student, when Hahnemann University was a homeopathic institution, I studied homeopathy with Dr. Boercke. To this day, I use homeopathy and belong to the National Center for Homeopathy. I attend the annual Florida Homeopath Conference. I attended Dr. Milton Erickson's hypnosis workshops. He taught me that we have all the resources we need within us and the unconscious is spontaneous, automatic, and creative. All action takes place in the unconscious. Communicate your ideas to the unconscious.

I model Dr. Candice Pert because she introduced us to the neuropeptides. The trillions of cells in our bodies communicate with each other by neuropeptides. She defines the mind as a form of energy in the mind-body.

Finally, I model Dr. Bruce Lipton, whom I met at a behavior conference. He is a famous molecular biologist who wrote a book on the biology of belief. He believes that the environment is more important than genes.

A healthy environment strengthens cell membranes, and environmental pollution damages cell membranes.

CHAPTER 1
The Many Faces of Relaxation

What is relaxation? According to the Tao, "relaxation" means total peace. One should return to the relaxed state on a regular basis. Relaxation simply renews us, purifies us, and leaves us with a profound state of serenity and tranquility. It is a wonderful state, away from problems. Relaxation is letting go of tension. Tighten your fist and let go completely.

Diaphragmatic breathing, or abdominal breathing, is most relaxing. Focus on your abdomen and breathe through your nose; inhale and allow your abdomen to rise. The diaphragm falls; exhale and allow your abdomen to fall, then your diaphragm rises.

All babies breathe abdominally. It is a natural technique.

When under stress, you breathe with your chest, very rapidly. When relaxed, you breathe slowly and regularly.

Let us talk about people who have contributed to physical relaxation. In 1920, a French pharmacist, Emile Coue, came up with a famous aphorism that became all the rage in Europe: "Day by day in every way, I am doing better and better. Day by day, I am more and more relaxed in every way."

My favorite technique for deep relaxation is the "5 to 1." Take a deep breath through the nose and count down from 5 to 1; with each decreasing number, become more and more deeply relaxed.

Take a deep breath though the nose and count on the out-breath 5, deeply relaxed; the deep breath 4, deeply, deeply relaxed; then deep breath 3, deeply relaxed; deep breath 2, deeply relaxed; then deep breath 1, at the bottom, the basement of relaxation.

Dr. Schultz, a German psychiatrist in 1880, developed autogenic therapy: "My arms and legs are heavy and warm. My arms and legs are numb, my heartbeat is calm and regular, my breathing is free and easy, my abdomen is warm, my forehead is cool, my mind is quiet and still."

Using these techniques, I can regress and relive my days in grade school. In 1933, I was a student in the Edgar Allan Poe Elementary School in Philadelphia. I was twelve years old, and my teacher was Mrs. Weiss, who was friendly and compassionate. I enjoyed her class very much. The school was located in South Philadelphia, at Twenty-Second and Ritner Streets.

I am now seated in the classroom; in front of me is the blackboard, with the alphabet on top and a tray at the bottom with a piece of white chalk. I pick up the chalk and write on the blackboard as I say, "I can relax." I again pick up the white chalk and write as I say, "I will relax." Then I take the chalk and write on the blackboard as I say, "I am relaxed." The ultimate of relaxation is one thought, one idea, and one task.

I am now completely relaxed. I allow the relaxation to flow to the back of my head, forehead, face, and nose; I drop my chin. All tension melts away.

I allow the relaxation to flow to my neck, right shoulder, arm, forearm, hand, fingers, and into the air.

I allow the relaxation to flow to my left shoulder, arm, forearm, hand, fingers, and into the air.

I allow the relaxation to flow to my chest and in between my ribs. Next, the relaxation flows to my abdomen.

Now, the warm relaxation flows to my right hip, thigh, patella, front of my legs, back of my legs, and the Achilles' tendon. Relaxation flows to my left hip, thigh, patella, front of my legs, back of my legs, and the Achilles' tendon.

In a moment, this warm relaxation flows from the top of my head to the tips of my toes. My entire body is encapsulated in a warm blanket of relaxation. All my muscles are completely relaxed.

Thoughts for a better, longer, and healthier life:

My brain is involved in everything I do. It weighs three pounds. My brain is electrical and has the electricity of a 25-watt bulb. The cranial electrotherapy stimulation (CES) of the brain is powered by 9 volts. Every morning I attach the electrodes with the felt pads to each ear. I stimulate my brain for twenty minutes.

The alpha stimulation causes a profound state of relaxation: the brain waves may go from alpha to theta waves. In addition to the deep relaxation, the CES takes care of depression and insomnia. I can do the electrotherapy stimulation of the brain for up to one hour. I enjoy this deep state of relaxation; when the electrodes are removed from my ears, the relaxation remains.

CHAPTER 2

On Becoming a Millionaire

I want to make a difference (one of my values).

I want to give everything that people want and get what I want; this is the golden rule in action.

When I do the things that I love and I do a good job, people appreciate it. When I do the things I love, I have happiness, joy, and peace of mind. If the thoughts, words, and actions as input are positive, the output is positive.

You must be before you can do, and do before you can have. If I am being abundant, and open the door to abundance and money, and do things that make money, I end up having peace of mind and happiness.

Abundance is everywhere in nature, in the fields, air, sky; it is also in relationships and friends.

I can create money by developing different strategies and using them, such as real estate, stocks, covered call options, hedge funds, fixed annuities, index annuities; I can also earn money by lecturing on health and counseling on psychological and physiological problems. I enjoy helping people and generously giving of my time—to give is to receive. If I contribute, I will be rewarded many times.

Let us talk about compound interest. Money is made by compounding it. If you take one dollar and compound it daily, in twenty days you will have one million dollars.

How long does it take to double your money? The rule of 72. The higher the interest rate, the less time it takes to double your money.

For example, a 10 percent interest rate divided by 72 equals 7 years to double your money; 6 percent divided by 72 equals 12 years; 2 percent divided by 72 equals 36 years; 20 percent divided by 72 equals 3 years plus; 8 percent divided by 72 equals 9 years.

If you want to be a millionaire in four years, you would have to put away and keep $250,000 a year. Pay yourself $250 an hour, according to Dr. Kappas (*Success Is Not an Accident*); identify your goals, prepare, and plan; list the benefits and the obstacles; and set a specific date that you expect to have the money.

Harvard University did a study to see how many people are independently wealthy by age sixty-five. The answer? Only 2 percent. The study revealed that those who were independently wealthy by age sixty-five all followed the habit of paying yourself first.

CHAPTER 3

Hypno-Birthing

I first learned self-hypnosis in 1968, when I took a six-month course at the University of Pennsylvania, and I have been teaching self-hypnosis for forty years. I used self-hypnosis in my general practice of internal medicine.

Every woman who enters the delivery room can be helped by hypnosis, and many can have complete freedom from discomfort. I believe that the ideal time for conditioning the patient is about the sixth month.

I give this kind of talk to expectant mothers: you are here for a very important reason, so that you can have your baby without feeling a thing, so you can have your baby with a great big smile on your face, so that you won't feel a thing, and so that the delivery of your baby will be a wonderful experience.

There is only one thing that will interfere with a pain-free delivery, and that is fear. Fear causes insecurity; everyone needs and wants to be secure. Fear immobilizes; when you are relaxed, you can't experience fear.

You may wonder, what is hypnosis? All hypnosis is self-hypnosis. There are many definitions for hypnosis. In the late 1800s, Dr. Bernheim called it "heightened suggestion." Some say it is a communication of ideas to the unconscious. The definition I like is this: hypnosis is a state of mind whereby you bypass the critical factor and replace it with selective thinking. The selective thinking can be a suggestion that you will not feel any pain.

When the time comes, you will have been conditioned for a pain-free delivery. At the time of delivery, you must be absolutely free of fear and worry. There should be only one thought on your mind: that in a little while, you are going to see your baby—the baby you have been waiting for.

If anything is bothering you, you should tell me about it. Is it possible that you won't get the state that we're working for now? I don't know; that is up to you. You must give your consent and follow the instructions. If you have to go to the bathroom, go now. All right, we will now get started. Please follow my instructions, and you will have a wonderful experience ahead of you.

Now the doctor or midwife can begin preparing the patient for hypnotic delivery. This can be done individually or with a group of women. The patients must be led into true somnambulism, otherwise the instructions that follow will be ineffective. It is only in true somnambulism that the patient will accept these suggestions.

There are three parts to the process: eye lock, relaxation, and numerical amnesia. In somnambulism, we have both physical and mental relaxation. The induction is as follows: "Now take a long deep breath and hold it for a few seconds. As you exhale this breath, allow your eyes to close. Just let your body relax as much as possible right now.

"Now, place your awareness on your eye muscles and relax the eye muscles around your eyes to the point that they won't work. Now when you are sure that they won't work, then test them to make sure that they won't work. When you test them, with your eyes closed, allow your eyelashes to go up and down three times; just let this quality of relaxation flow through your whole body, from the top of your head to the tips of your toes. Now we can deepen this relaxation much more.

"In a moment, I am going to have you open and close your eyes and allow the warm relaxation to flow from the top of your head to the tips of your toes. Now open and close your eyes and allow that warm relaxation to flow from the top of your head to the tips of your toes; double the relaxation. Now, once more allow the warm relaxation to flow from the top of your head to the tips of your toes. Double the relaxation once again. Each time you do this, you will do better and better. Let us test the relaxation. In a moment, I am going to lift your hand by the wrist just a few inches and drop it, and it will plop down. Let me do the lifting.

"You have already proved that you can relax physically, now let me show you how to relax mentally. In a moment, I am going to ask you to begin slowly counting backwards, out loud, from 100. With each number you say, let your mind become twice as relaxed. Now if you do this, by the time you reach 98 or less, you will have relaxed all the rest of the numbers out of your mind.

"Now, say the first number, 100, and double your mental relaxation. The numbers are fading, disappearing; 99, twice as relaxed, all gone, lights out. They are completely gone.

"Now I want to tell you the benefits of relaxation. You know very well that if you were tense and I had to give you an injection, you would feel the entrance of the needle very sharply because of the fact that you were tense, wouldn't you? If you were completely relaxed, you would not feel the entrance of the needle. You can reach such a state of relaxation so that you have no discomfort at all at the time of delivery. It is in this state when you are physically and mentally relaxed that it is so easy to have a baby. It is in this state that the contractions, or surges, instead of being unpleasant, become very pleasant."

The average mother-to-be has heard talk from friends or relatives that having a baby is a terrible ordeal. So she looks forward to what she has heard described as labor, labor pains, or hard labor. There is no such thing as labor, labor pains, or hard labor.

But we can change that to the right attitude by explaining to patients just what happens when a baby is born. Nature has a method of making the birth of a baby possible by contractions. In the uterus, there are circular and longitudinal muscles that push the baby forward (similarly, in the intestines, there are circular and longitudinal muscles that push the food forward). Peristalsis is a wave of contraction, followed by a wave of relaxation. The longitudinal muscles in the uterus contract, and push the baby forward so the baby can be born very easily. In the first stage of labor, there are contractions and relaxation. With hypnosis, there are still contractions, but you don't have labor pains or hard labor.

And the odd thing about these contractions is that if you look forward to them pleasantly and know that they are going to be something nice to have, you won't mind them at all. I will be there to help you with the birth of the baby, but until I get there, I want you to relax as you are relaxed now. One of the wonderful things this relaxation will do is to shorten the delivery period tremendously. It can shorten the delivery time by as much as three hours. With each contraction, you will feel more and more relaxed. By the third or fourth contraction, you will be smiling and looking forward to the next one, as you say, "I am much closer to the birth of my baby."

Remember that this relaxation that you are feeling now is going to be used in addition to all the aids that medical science has invented, such as caudal anesthesia and nitrous oxide (nitrous oxide is sometimes used when there is complete dilatation of the cervix and the baby's head is pushing into the dilated vagina).

After the baby is born, you will feel so good. A few minutes after the birth of the baby, you will be able to use the telephone to call your friends. You will be just as strong then as you are now. Your strength will be complete, your feeling of well-being will be complete, and you will recover much more quickly than you ordinarily would. Then if you want to nurse your baby, this relaxation will make it possible for you to do so very, very easily.

I want you to practice relaxation, just as you are doing now. Learn how to relax at home, so when your baby comes, you will be all ready for it; you will feel so wonderful on the day of delivery, during the delivery, and after the delivery. Notice how the feeling of relaxation holds on and makes you say to yourself, "Motherhood is going to be a glorious adventure for me. I'm going to love every minute of it."

Dr. Milton Erickson's hand levitation is one way to numb the jaw and produce dental anesthesia. Place your right hand on your lap and, with your left hand, raise your right hand and allow it to rise toward your face; with each breath, the hand will rise higher and higher. Sometimes I attach a balloon to my wrist to speed up the ascent to my face and jaw. When my right hand reaches my jaw, I will be twice as relaxed and my jaw will be twice as numb, then ten times as numb, just as if I was injected with Novocain. My jaw is now numb, and I stroke my jaw three times and take the numbness and transfer it to my abdomen. This numbness in my hand is referred to as glove anesthesia. I can numb a patient's uterus by transferring the numbness to the abdomen by stroking it three times, and pressing on the abdomen with my right hand. Dr. Bill Kroger, an obstetrician, uses glove anesthesia to numb the uterus, vagina, and perineum.

Once you have produced numbness, you can transfer it to any part of your body. The numbness will neutralize discomfort in any part of your body, so that you will hardly feel anything. Remember, your right hand will carry and transfer the numbness wherever you need it.

CHAPTER 4

Health and Healing

Love is the foundation of healing. Healing depends on healthy perceptions, healthy attitudes, and a healthy lifestyle. See yourself as already healed, believe it, and achieve it. Imagine and feel yourself as already healed, believe it, and achieve it. Remember, the body heals itself. A healthy attitude and mental posture makes for healing. See yourself as loving, capable, and worthwhile. A healthy lifestyle means avoiding smoking, alcohol, sugar, caffeine, dairy products, and red meat. Encourage the habit of exercise, and hope for a better future. Besides love and compassion, balance is a major component of healing, particularly psychological and physiological balance. Remember, genetics and environmental factors can interfere with healing and produce an imbalance and disease.

The revelation of wholeness, the unification of the mind, heart, and spirit as one, is key. You don't have to do anything to heal. Embrace silence, do nothing, just be. Be a silent witness to your thoughts, impulses of intelligence, and your breathing. The healing will take place automatically. Your unconscious has all the resources you need.

You are consciousness and pure potential. Your spirit is pure potential energy, which you can tap into with empowering beliefs and attitudes, and move the energy into action, which gets a result (which can be good or bad), and we can keep changing until we get the desired result.

Your subconscious is automatic, spontaneous, and creative; it is the doer. All the action and creativity takes place in the subconscious. The soul is the thinker of thoughts and is the creator. The soul creates the body and the ego personality. The ego personality is impermanent, while the soul is permanent. The ego personality is destructive, with negative low-energy thoughts such as anger, fear, hate, resentment, anxiety, guilt, shame, and blame. The soul has the higher energy thoughts of love, joy, peace, and forgiveness. The goal of enlightenment is the integration of the personality with the soul. The aim is to release the ego and the self and become the no-self (egoless).

There is a psychological solution to all our problems; Wayne Dyer encourages us to stay connected to our source, our spirit. When we separate from our source, the destructive ego becomes powerful; according to A Course in Miracles, there are no problems, we only think that we have problems. If we change our mind, our thoughts (impulses of intelligence), we eliminate our problems. The amazing thing is that we have control of our minds; we can change our mind at any time. The mind and body are within us. In fact, the universe is within is. Human awareness and the cosmic consciousness are one. Our true self is within the silent space between our thoughts. Our thoughts come from the gap, the light, between our thoughts. In this space is our insight, choices, potentiality, universal mind, and God. This space connects to immortality and eternity. We have within us the atoms of all great men and women of history, like Albert Schweitzer, Albert Einstein, Thomas Edison, Thomas Jefferson, Catherine the Great, Florence Nightingale, and Joan of Arc. Insights are inner visions of life without words; it is an inner knowing, and the words come later. When we speak, the words have less meaning than body language and tonality.

Health is a state of physical, mental, emotional, and spiritual well-being. We have to be, before we can do, and do, before we can have. See yourself as whole, healthy, strong, and vital. Do healthy activities; follow a healthy Mediterranean diet; develop a healthy lifestyle, with a focus on nutrition, exercise, meditation, and self-hypnosis, and you will have peace of mind and happiness.

An imbalance and a lack of love and compassion cause illness, disease, and death. Just as a healthy lifestyle and attitude cause balance, wholeness, and healing, an unhealthy lifestyle causes imbalance, disease, and symptoms. Disease needs the services of a doctor; healing only needs yourself, regulation, and personal care.

CHAPTER 5

Smoking Cessation

Monica is a heavy smoker; she smokes one and a half to two packs of cigarettes a day. She has been smoking for many years and is a heavy coffee drinker. On the positive side, she walks one to two miles daily and belongs to a gym; she works out three times a week.

I tell Monica she is loveable, capable, and worthwhile. Monica would like to relax and be calm and confident without cigarettes. I suggest she use the following exercise, which I have learned from Dr. Cory Hammond at Utah University to help people relax and stop smoking.

"Place your right thumb and index finger together and take a deep breath through your nose. Count down from 5 to 1, and with each count down, you will become more and more relaxed. This is called the 5 to 1 countdown. Take a deep breath through your nose and with the fifth out-breath, deeply relax; take a deep breath through your nose and with the fourth out-breath, deeply relax; take a deep breath through your nose and with the third out-breath, deeply relax; take a deep breath through your nose and with the second out-breath, deeply relax; pause. Now, breathe through your nose deeply; relax the bottom of relaxation, the basement; pause now; you see yourself as relaxed, calm, cool, and confident. Whatever you conceive, believe you can achieve.

"Now you are the new Monica, the birth of a new life. A new Monica. Now, say to yourself, 'I see smoking as a poison for my body; I need my body to live. I owe my body respect and protection. I now release myself from the itching to smoke, and the itch will get smaller and smaller and vanish in thin air. I see myself in control, masterfully meeting the situation head on with confidence, success, and the winning way.'" In addition to relaxation, wellness is important. Wellness depends on a healthy diet, lifestyle, nutrition, exercise, and mind-body connection. Remember, the body heals itself; Dr. Schweitzer said there is doctor inside each of us.

Monica is a success story. She stopped smoking for more than ten years, got married, and moved out of state with her husband. She has a very happy marriage.

I would like to leave you with these thoughts:

Every moment of love,
every moment of giving,
every moment of joy,
is a moment of living.

CHAPTER 6
Buddhism

The essence of Buddhist teaching can be summed up in the following: Keep your mind open to all possibilities and attach yourself to nothing. When you don't attach to anything, you are free. Nothing is worth holding onto. If you let go of everything—objects, concepts, teachers, Buddha, self, senses, memories, life, death, freedom—all suffering will cease. The world will appear in its pristine nature, and you will experience the freedom of the Buddha. See yourself as pure energy, with all the subtleties of consciousness. After all, we are pure potentiality and consciousness (or awareness).

According to Eastern thought, violence, suffering, and illness are due to judging and grasping at self. When we are too attached to our ego, the destructive ego, we have problems.

Our false self, our destructive ego, is of low energy and vibration. It is wise to free ourselves from anger, fear, anxiety, and depression. Replace the past, guilt, shame, and blame, with a higher energy of love, joy, peace, and forgiveness.

We must tame our ego and remain connected to the source. How do we release ourselves from grasping at the self? By embracing silence; being nonjudgmental; and having moment-to-moment awareness, mindfulness, compassion, devotion, and pure perception. When we release our self and become no-self, or egoless, we tap into the silent gap between thoughts, where our insight, choice, and higher self (or true self) are located. Our true self is the immortal soul.

When we die, we join and connect to the soul; it was Plato who coined the term "immortal soul." He used the Socratic method to explain morality and knowledge.

It is very important to stay connected to the spirit, the source. There is a spiritual solution to our problems. All we need to do is embrace silence and meditate, and answers to our problems will come.

Buddhism is based on the four noble truths:

1. In every life there is suffering.
2. The cause of suffering is desire, greed, delusion; the desire for something we do not have, the desire for things to be different from how they are at this moment.
3. The pathway to the relief of suffering is the extinguishing of desire.
4. There is a pathway to follow that will lead to the release of desire.

Buddhism suggests that we live our entire lives developing the qualities of acceptance and compassion, continually releasing our attachment to things, people, and ideas. We can learn to relax by mindfulness meditation twenty to thirty minutes every morning and evening.

CHAPTER 7

Alcohol Addiction

Alcoholism is a symptom of a deep-seated personality disorder, usually selected to avoid an intolerable situation. Alcoholism is an addiction, a permanent, impulsive craving to drink.

Alcoholism is both an addiction and a personality disorder with physiological complications; the complications are fatty infiltration of the liver, hepatic cirrhosis, brain damage, pancreatitis, neuropathy, and anxiety or depression. You need to say to yourself, "Alcohol is a poison for my body. I need my body to live. I owe my body respect and protection."

What is the personality profile of the person with a drinking addiction? The alcoholic has feelings of inadequacy, insecurity, shyness, anxiety, panic, and anger. There is an emotional conflict and a need for self-punishment. There is also a conflict and imbalance between drinking and nondrinking.

If you drink, there is a temporary euphoria, followed by anxiety and depression. The anxiety at times is unbearable. If you don't drink, you have an impulsive craving to drink; you think about the pleasurable feeling of drinking; others drink to drown out their feelings of unworthiness. You are caught between a rock and a hard place, and the only solution is love and support, like that of the AA program.

You may regress to childish behavior and have a need for instant oral gratification. You may even regress to an infantile behavior, to be held in your mother's arms, receiving the touch and love of a mother.

Many alcoholics never emerge from adolescence, the undifferentiated period of psychosexual development, which is characteristic of homosexual tendencies. The alcohol serves the purpose of fending off the homosexual drives (panic).

By using self-hypnosis, you can bypass the critical judgment, the analytical, verbal, suggestive part of your mind, and replace it with selective thinking or awareness. For the alcoholic, there is no room for criticism or blaming; you are a loving, capable, worthwhile human being who treasures her divinity. There is a piece of God within you.

The objective mind is only analytical. It does nothing but analyze and compare. The subconscious is automatic, spontaneous, and creative. All the action takes place in the subconscious, where the spirit, soul, and God are. Our thoughts arise from the silent gap between thoughts. The gap is where the light, the universal mind, is hidden.

The Addiction Cycle

One of the most virulent of these is the addiction cycle. Picture a child at the crest of a hill, fashioning a large, icy snowball. He checks the fall line, makes sure there are no rocks or trees in the way, and pushes the snowball down the long hill. Clunky and uncertain at first, the snowball slowly picks up weight, speed, momentum. Halfway down, it has already burgeoned into a Godzilla of a monster, mindless and unstoppable. By the time it reaches the bottom, it has become the snowball of death. The addiction cycle is that snowball.

At first, counselors assumed codependency was strictly an effect, a syndrome in people who lived closely with alcoholics and other addicts. Now we see that regardless of what launched your codependency, once the condition is in place, the addiction cycle both perpetuates and amplifies it. It now maintains its own internal, addictive momentum. No longer can you ease codependency simply by identifying and dealing with the cause. You must do that, but you must also take definite steps to recover from the codependency itself, and you must break the addiction component that feeds it.

The Mechanics of the Addiction Cycle

Our view of the addiction cycle comes from the old classic model used by counselors and researchers studying alcohol and drug addiction. In that model, usually described as a spiraling circle, the subject feels pain of some sort, low self-esteem, guilt, dissatisfaction, pressure, or simply the sheer boredom life can bring. He finds anesthesia in alcohol or drugs, but getting drunk or high creates consequences: remorse, greater guilt, even more pain. The subject found relief once in his anesthetic, so he returns to it. The consequences increase to include depression, loss of health, perhaps even the loss of job and family, leading to more guilt and shame, more remorse, more anesthetic.

In treating an addicted patient, whom I will call Rosemarie, I used the following images:

Just as the butterfly emerges from the cocoon, love emerges from the wings of forgiveness.

Rosemarie, because you are now clean, you can say to yourself the following:

I am a problem drinker.
I am now clean.
I am no longer powerless.
I now have a choice to drink or not to drink.
I do not have an incurable disease.
I am in control.
I am no longer neurotic and psychotic.
I believe that I have within me a divine white light.
I have a spiritual and soul energy within.
I have decided to use this higher energy to solve my problems
I make a list of my successes, not my failures.
I can learn from my mistakes and grow.
I know there is no failure, only learning and changing.
I am taking full responsibility, without blaming others.
I am now successful.
I have a job, I am helping others, and I am paying my debts.
I release all resentment, guilt, anger, shame, and negativity.
I now follow a path of forgiveness and love.
Before I go to bed, I pray to Jesus and say I forgive myself for my mistakes and forgive others whom I think have wronged me.
I am good enough.
I am no longer unworthy.
I am somebody.
I am love.

What is the secret of being clean and free from alcohol? The secret is to love yourself and take responsibility for your life.

The higher the self-esteem, the less the need for alcohol. Enjoy life without the alcohol. The alcoholic person thinks, "In the past, every time I had a problem the only solution I knew was to drink alcohol. I thought the alcohol would make me feel better, but in time the alcohol made me nervous and depressed, at times leading to thoughts of suicide. Now, the hopelessness is gone forever. I know now that I cannot drink alcohol. I must abstain from alcohol completely."

Successfully treated alcoholics know that they are good enough and can face the world with self-confidence. They say, "Now there are greater things ahead for me. I have the ability to create new things in the computer field. I truly can enjoy my life without the alcohol as the self-esteem grows bigger and bigger, the need for alcohol grows smaller and smaller and eventually disappears completely."

CHAPTER 8

Fear and Love

Two important emotions are fear and love. We usually fear something, like the fear of public speaking, the fear of social contact, or the fear of authority. There are also irrational fears that seem to come from nowhere. They are imaginary fears that something dreadful is going to happen to you, or you are going to have a heart attack. Fear paralyzes us and inhibits performance. For example, when you are taking an examination, along comes fear, and it interferes with the exam and you do poorly and your immune system also suffers. What can you do?

You can rehearse for the exam and be prepared; see yourself being relaxed, calm, and confident. Believe it and achieve it. Whatever you conceive, believe you can achieve. Love yourself and accept yourself. Love overcomes fear. You can embrace silence, meditate, or do self-hypnosis. It is not what is in front of you or behind you, but what is inside of you. Your unconscious is automatic, spontaneous, and creative, while your conscious mind or willpower is only analytical, verbal, and suggestive. It does nothing. It passes on suggestions to the unconscious, which unequivocally accepts them and carries them out. All the action, all the resources are in the unconscious. Learn to tap into the universal mind, which is in the unconscious, where the spirit and the soul are also located.

It is rare to have depression without anxiety. To help anxiety, I have prescribed antidepressants like Lexopro (20 mg in the morning) and Trazadone (50 mg at bedtime). The Trazadone allows the patient to go to sleep quickly and awaken in the morning refreshed, without any side effects.

The nonpharmacological approach to anxiety is self-hypnosis. In my practice, I use the body scan and do relaxation exercises, progressively relaxing all the muscles in the body, followed by exercises to enhance the self-esteem. In the Western world, lack of self-esteem is a real problem, while Eastern countries do not have this problem.

The Dalai Lama feels that it is natural to love oneself and others, to give loving kindness to ourselves and spread it to the whole world. The Dalai Lama believes that the purpose in life is to be happy and have peace of mind.

I also believe that a major goal in life is peace of mind and that fear is the biggest obstacle in reaching that goal, along with a low self-image. We are all here on this planet for a purpose. My purpose is to learn and teach. I also want harmonious relationships and to have friends and hope for a better future; of course, financial security is also important.

The main problem in Western society is feeling that one is not good enough, unworthy. We must learn to love ourselves. Another exercise that I like is the mirror exercise, which I learned from Louise Hay. Look in the mirror each morning and say, "I love myself, therefore I feel better. I love myself, therefore I can think, feel, and behave better. I love myself, therefore I take care of my body, my home, my spouse, my children. I am loving, capable, and worthwhile. If I have love inside of me, that is what I give out. If I have hate inside of me, that is what I give out. If I give service to others, I am rewarded manyfold."

Anxiety causes stress and a release of adrenalin due to a stimulation of the sympathetic nervous system. There is rapid irregular breathing, a rapid heart rate, an increase in blood pressure (BP), blood clots, an increase in blood sugar, and increased muscle tension. Hypnosis and meditation slow the breathing and make it regular. The heart rate and blood pressure come down; the anxious person may have palpitations, hyperventilation, queasy stomach, headache, and so on. Learn to breathe through your nose and count from 5 to 1; with each count, become more and more relaxed. Use deep relaxation and visual imagery. See yourself confronting the situation with success, confidence, and the winning way.

I leave you with my favorite poem:

Every moment of love,
Every moment of giving,
Every moment of joy,
Is a moment of living.
Every moment of anger,

Every moment of lying,
Every moment of fear,
Is a moment of dying.
You have a choice to live or die.

Success is love, joy, and peace. Love is giving each other a higher positive energy, so as to nurture and nourish each soul. Happiness is thinking pleasant thoughts.

CHAPTER 9
Change

If you keep doing the same thing, you keep getting the same result. Everything in the universe is changing. Existence is impermanent, unsatisfactory, and empty.

The destructive ego is part of the emptiness and lack of sustainability. Our destructive ego personality is our anger, fear, resentment, guilt, anxiety, shame, and blame. These emotions are of low energy, frequency, and vibration, while love, joy, and peace are of higher energy and represent success.

The universe is nothing more than energy, motion, and change. The sky and the sun are changing; the ocean is changing—one time it is turbulent, another time it is placid and tranquil. Even though the ocean may be rough and turbulent, the bottom of the ocean may be quiet, silent, and peaceful. When the sun rises in the morning, it may be orange or red in color; it may change to golden yellow or white. Change is everywhere, but we humans resist change. We fear leaving the comfort zone. We resist change because of fear and low self-image. We need to release ourselves from the need to resist change. We can release ourselves from the chains of the past and the prison of guilt. Forgiveness is the path of love; just as the butterfly emerges from the cocoon, love emerges from the wings of forgiveness. Learn to forgive ourselves and others. Release all the low energy emotions such as anger, fear, and resentment and replace these afflictive emotions with the higher energy, higher frequency emotions such as love, joy, and peace.

We have control of our mind, and we can change our thoughts anytime we want to do so. According to A Course in Miracles, there are no problems; we only think that we have problems. If we change our mind, we can eliminate the problems. We can control our thoughts. Thoughts create our future.

The thoughts of today create the body of tomorrow. Action and feeling follow our thoughts. Action is followed by a result, which could be good or bad. And we can always keep changing until we get a desirable result.

The mitochondria are burners present in each cell. CoQ10 not only burns fats but also glucose, increasing energy and activating the universal energizer, adenyl triphosphate.

The Mediterranean diet consists of grains, oatmeal, brown rice, spelt and Jerusalem artichoke pasta (regular pasta has too much carbs), veggies, fruits. Five veggies and three fruits daily, beans, nuts, and cold-water fish. Chicken and turkey are permitted. Avoid red meat and dairy products.

Garlic lowers BP and cholesterol because of the chemical allicin, and onions lower BP because of quercertin. The body is composed of 70 to 80 percent water; all the cells in the body need water. Drink an eight-ounce glass of clean water every hour or eight to ten glasses of water daily.

A healthy lifestyle means avoiding smoking, alcohol, and caffeine. As we have mentioned, the cruciferous green veggies supply the body with calcium, vitamin E, potassium, and folic acid. These vegetables include cabbage, broccoli, Brussels sprouts, spinach, kale, and cauliflower. These veggies lower the BP and also help patients with breast cancer by supplying Indole 3 Carbinol.

Folic acid is also found in asparagus. It strengthens the heart and prevents hardening of the arteries and atherosclerosis. Folic acid, B12, and B6 prevent the elevation of homocysteine, which can cause heart attacks. I believe an increase in homocysteine is a bigger cause of heart attacks than cholesterol. Cantaloupe supplies beta-carotene, and grape fruit, berries, strawberries, apples, and pears supply vitamin C.

As a morning cereal, oatmeal (not instant) is by far the best because it supplies water-soluble fiber (beta glucan). It is very difficult to get five veggies and three fruits on a daily basis. I personally like to juice; I own a Juiceman. I juice apples, carrots, cabbage, broccoli, and strawberries. I add three teaspoonfuls of Superfoods Greens Plus and one half ounce of New Vitality's 18X Aloe Vera (you could use other aloe vera juice). You could add a banana and make a smoothie. There are many variations; you can add different vegetables and fruits. I also take antioxidants to neutralize the free radicals, which cause heart disease and other degenerative diseases. I think it is necessary to take nutritional supplements.

Fifty million people suffer from high blood pressure, and over 38,000 die every year.

CHAPTER 10

Letting Go of Resentment—Dedicated to Mary McNamara

I am no longer chained to resentment of the past or imprisoned by guilt. I release myself from resentment. I allow guilt and fear to fly from the palm of my hand and float into the sky and disappear. The palm of my hand is now full of loving kindness. My being is love, I do things that bring forth loving kindness, and I have happiness and peace of mind.

Just as the butterfly emerges from the cocoon, love emerges from the wings of forgiveness. Guilt, fear, and negativity are released when you follow the path of forgiveness, for they are replaced with love, joy, and peace. The foundation of all healing is love and forgiveness.

Jesus is love, and in the Lord's Prayer, he tells us to forgive ourselves for our mistakes, and forgive others whom we think have wronged us ("forgive us our trespasses as we forgive those who have trespassed against us"). Before you go to bed, pray to Jesus and say, "I forgive myself for my mistakes, and I forgive others who I think have wronged me." When you forgive, love emerges.

Remember the Prayer of St. Francis: "Make me an instrument of your peace. Where there is hate, let there be love; where there is despair, let there be hope; where there is hurt, let there be pardon; where there is doubt, let there be faith; where there is darkness, let there be light; where there is sadness, let there be joy."

CHAPTER 11

On Asthma, Hypertension, and Healing Chronic Back Pain

Asthma is caused by spasms of the smaller bronchioles of the lung. Tension prevents the release of air in exhalation, resulting in wheezing and shortness of breath. Deep relaxation and visual imagery reduces the tension in the smooth muscle of the bronchioles, allowing the escape of air and relief of wheezing and dyspnea. Acute asthma is an overactivity of the immune system and hypersensitivity due to pollen, dander, and stress. Very stressful situations can trigger asthma.

In hypertension, the smaller arteriolar vessels are constricted and spastic. Internal stressors such as anxiety, anger, fear, and resentment can stimulate the sympathetic nervous system with a release of adrenalin and an increase in heart rate and blood pressure.

When there is an imbalance of the autonomic nervous system, the flight-or-fight mechanism comes into play. Our ancestors had to fight animals or run away in order to survive. Modern man does not fight or run away; instead, he bears the brunt of the stress.

How Do We Handle Discomfort?

1. Education: One must become aware of the mechanisms behind tension and muscular spasm, and the unconscious factors: emotion and repressed anger.
2. Use relaxing mental exercises.
3. Distraction: Move away from pain toward pleasure, learn how to use pain and pleasure.
4. Dissociation: Produce numbness, warmth, and coldness in the hands and transfer the numbness to other parts of the body. This requires daily condition and practice with mental rehearsing. Use Ericksonian hand levitation for relaxation and

numbness. Then transfer the numbness to the jaw, hand, neck, back, and any area that is needed. Use a row of colored lights in order to control the electrical impulses. For example, select the blue light, which is connected to the hand. Shut off the blue light and the power to the right hand is cut out; the right hand falls asleep and becomes numb. The hand is dissociated and hardly feels anything. It is no longer part of you. You can then transfer the numbness to other parts of the body.

Chronic back pain, which can last for years, can be caused by tension, muscle spasm, inflammation, and ischemia (oxygen deprivation). Back pain is associated with tenderness.

The vicious cycle of discomfort and muscle spasm is triggered by anxiety and anger, particularly repressed anger. Repressed anger is in the unconscious, out of awareness, and is manifested by back, buttock, neck, and shoulder pain. Long-standing back pain is emotional and not structural. It is not due to disc or arthritis problems.

Negative thoughts can trigger anger. Impatience can trigger anger. Be patient, relaxed, calm, and confident. Fill yourself with loving kindness and spread it to others, and the anger will be dispelled. Anger stored in the unconscious plays a big part in the manifestation of chronic back pain.

The repressed anger, anxiety, and apprehension cause tension and muscle spasms. When the muscles are deeply relaxed, there is no tension and discomfort. There is only comfort.

Fibromyalgia (fibrositis) is due to tension and muscle spasm and is predominantly emotional. Multiple muscles are involved with tenderness. Fatigue and exhaustion are due to the stress hormone cortisol.

The muscles involved are the back, buttock, hip, neck, shoulder, and top of shoulder. Many psychosomatic diseases are due to tension: muscular spasms, tension headaches, migraine headaches, irritable bowels, asthma, and hypertension, to name a few. Tension headaches are caused by skeletal muscle spasms and tension of the neck muscles.

Migraines involve spasms (constriction), dilation, and edema of the temporal vessels; warming of the hands releases the constriction, while cold constricts the dilation and takes away the pain.

Irritable bowel is caused by muscle tension and muscle spasm of the left side of the colon, sigmoid, and descending colon; the patient complains of constipation, diarrhea, and diarrhea alternating with constipation. There is tenderness to palpation. Deep relaxation and visual imagery release the tension and spasm. When there is relaxation, there is no tension.

Chapter 12
Obesity

There is an epidemic of obesity in the United States. Obesity breeds heart disease, hypertension, hypercholesteremia, diabetes, and even cancer. Overweight people are prone to osteoporosis. We see more and more obesity and diabetes among the youth of America. In 1999, there were approximately 100 million people in the United States that were overweight or obese, according to the *AMA Journal.*

We are a nation of couch potatoes and spend too much time watching TV. What can we do about this problem? We must address this problem in four ways:

1. Diet and lifestyle
2. Nutritional supplements and weight reduction herbs
3. Exercise program and resistant exercises
4. Relaxation techniques

Start off with a low-fat diet; 20 percent of the total caloric intake should be calories, no more. The diet should emphasize complex carbs and high fiber. The ratio should be 50 percent complex carbohydrates, 30 percent protein, and 20 percent fats. We should have a clear understanding of the difference between complex and concentrated carbs.

Complex carbohydrates include grains such as oatmeal (complete, not instant), brown rice, spelt pasta, Jerusalem artichoke pasta, and durum wheat pasta. Avoid egg pasta and limit the regular durum wheat pastas.

A nutritious diet includes vegetables such as cabbage, Brussels sprouts, broccoli florets, and beans. Cabbage juice heals ulcers and contains Indole 3 Carbinol, which can protect against breast cancer. Many of these veggies supply magnesium, calcium, and potassium.

Steamed asparagus supplies folic acid, which can prevent atherosclerosis. Spinach contains lutein. Fruits are important, particularly berries and strawberries, apples and pears (for vitamin C), and melons (for beta-carotene). Beans and nuts wind up in the complex group. Beans have magnesium and potassium, are low in fat, and are high in fiber and protein. Beans include lentils, chickpeas, red kidney beans, and white beans. It is a good idea to take a carb with a protein.

Now, what is a concentrated carbohydrate? Sugar, cakes, donuts, pies, cookies, ice cream. When you take these sugars, there is an insulin surge along with the increase in blood sugar. The insulin goes into the blood stream and is transported to the liver, where it is converted to fat and triglycerides. We want a slow release of the carbs, aided by fiber, which prevents the insulin surge; the complex group does exactly that.

Learn to read nutritional labels. Take the total calories and divide it by the fat calories. If the answer is 5 or more, that means that the fat calories are 20 percent or less, and it is okay to use it. For example, if the label reads total calories 150 and the fat calories are 15, this would be 10 percent, and it is okay to use.

Lose weight slowly, about one pound a week. If your goal is twelve pounds, that should take twelve weeks. Do not rely on the scale; measure your waist and your body fat once a month.

Lifestyle is important. Avoid smoking, caffeine, sugar, red meat, dairy products, recreational drugs, and excessive use of alcohol. A healthy Mediterranean diet is important, as is exercise.

We have mentioned that a healthy diet includes grains, vegetables, fruits, beans, and nuts. For added protein, it is okay to add cold-water fish, which supply omega and CoQ10. Cold-water fish includes salmon, Atlantic halibut, snapper, cod, mackerel, sardines, and herring. Cold-water fish twice a week can prevent sudden cardiac death. Avoid red meat and dairy products, but consider the soy bean: soy milk, tofu, tempeh; miso supplies magnesium, potassium, and omega 3.

Nutritional supplements are also important. Take a multivitamin and mineral, as well as antioxidants. Take vitamins A, B, C, and E; CoQ10 and grape seed extract can also help. Specific nutrients for weight loss include the trace mineral chromium picolinate, which regulates blood sugar, insulin, and metabolism. The amino acid l-Carnitine transports fat from cells to the mitochondrium, where it is burned.

There are two Indian herbs that are extremely important for weight loss. Gymnema Silvestri cuts the appetite for sweets, and carcinia cambogia (hydroxyl citrate) prevents fat storage. Chromium picolinate should be used in doses of 200 to 600 mg (in some cases, 1000 mg). Free-range chicken and turkey can be added to the food program in addition to fish as a protein source.

The final and most important part of any weight loss program is exercise. Exercise five mornings a week. Start with aerobics, preferably walking briskly. Exercise for thirty minutes initially and increase to forty-five minutes. Walk a mile in fifteen minutes eventually. To establish your target heart rate, take 185 and subtract your age. If you are forty, then the target would be 145. Exercise increases cardiac output and vital capacity. It also raises HDL and increases growth hormone.

Anger
I am anger
I hide underneath impatience.
I am a monster with big ears and horns with a red face.
I attack joints and cause arthritis.
I run away from loving, joyous thoughts
I attack in the presence of harmful thoughts
I enjoy thoughts of enmity and allow them to spread and grow into unruly behavior
I cannot survive in the presence of love.
I manage anger by filling my being with loving kindness.

CHAPTER 13

How to Handle Pain

Anger is a slow, low vibrational energy; under the surface of impatience is anger. Enmity, hostility, animosity, and harmful thoughts trigger anger. There are no such things as problems; you only think you have problems. If you change your thoughts and feelings, you eliminate problems.

Perhaps someone has deflated my ego and spoke critically to me: "Look me in the eye when you talk to me; speak softly; you are disorganized; you don't process information properly; cut the hairs from your nose; you look sloppy. Speak so that I can understand you." If I view these statements as inflammatory and think harmful thoughts toward the person making them, this will trigger anger. If I dwell on these thoughts of enmity, the anger can grow and spread to the point of rage and unruly behavior, such as cursing the person and calling them nasty names.

Instead of harmful thoughts, if I think loving thoughts, along with patience, and say to the person, "You are right," there will be no anger. Anger cannot exist when there is loving thoughts. What I have done was change my mind, change my thoughts from harmful to loving. Problems are due to thoughts. Wisdom is avoiding the slow, low vibrational energies such as anger, fear, resentment, and hate and using the higher thought energies such as love, joy, peace, and happiness.

Happiness in nothing more than thinking pleasant thoughts most of the time. According to Einstein, the mind that creates a problem cannot solve it. It requires another mind, and change. For example, if my daughter is talking to me on the phone and disagrees with me, she may get angry and hang up on me. If I have thoughts of enmity and hostility, this would trigger anger, but if I have higher vibrational energy thoughts of love, I would not feel anger.

We have control of our mind, our thoughts, and our feelings. We can change our mind and eliminate all problems. The ego, the I and me, the materialistic world is where we have our harmful thoughts and our desire to get even. If we stay connected to our source, the spirit, love, compassion, there is no problem. The spirit is in the body and is the cause; the effect is the ego. The Dalai Lama does not understand low self-esteem. He believes that we can go from self, ego, to the no-self, the spirit; in the subjective unconscious, the spiritual energy, there is love, God, the universal mind. Life is impermanent, but God never changes. In the ego consciousness, there is change. The spirit, the soul is permanent, but the body and personality are always changing.

One way to treat pain is to eliminate the source. Many people have diverticulitis, a painful disease. Here is the treatment for diverticulitis of the sigmoid colon (out pocketings of the inner lining and the submucosa with abscess formation):

1. Do not eat red meat.
2. Take Superfoods Greens Plus twice a day; in the morning, take eight ounces of apple juice plus three teaspoonfuls of Greens Plus and one and a half ounces of aloe vera.
3. In the afternoon, take eight ounces of organic veggie juice and add three teaspoonfuls of Greens Plus.
4. You need 40 gm of soluble fiber daily; take two teaspoonfuls of enhanced fiber powder in juice or distilled water four times a day. Each teaspoonful has 5 gm of fiber.
5. Drink one glass of cold distilled water eight times a day.
6. Drink one cup of warm organic veggie broth three times a day.
7. Eat oatmeal in the morning.
8. Take Cipro antibiotic every twelve hours.
9. To prevent abnormal fungus growth in the intestines, take Metromidazole.
10. For the pain, take 10 mg of Ketoralac every four to six hours (stop after five days because it can cause ulcers if you take it longer).
11. Rest in bed.
12. Place a warm heating pad on the left lower abdomen.

CHAPTER 14
Wholeness and Oneness

When we feel at one with everything, we feel whole ourselves. When we are in touch with being whole, we feel at one with everything. Wholeness is the root of these words: healing, health, and holy. When we reconnect with our body and merge our breath with the universe, we experience ourselves as whole.

See yourself as whole, healthy, strong, and vital. Believe it and achieve it. Whatever you conceive, believe you can achieve. When I see myself as whole, I feel that I am one with everything.

Peace comes within the soul when you realize that you are one with the universe. Knowing our wholeness as we meditate brings us closer to who we are; wholeness and oneness give us a taste of our connection to each other; we are all connected in the material world, and there is no barrier between self and no-self.

Healing is influenced by thought and feelings. Healing depends on balance, harmony, and wholeness. A healthy attitude and lifestyle invites psychological and physiological balance and harmony. When we have an unhealthy attitude and lifestyle, we invite a mind and body imbalance, and disease. It is important to take responsibility for your health and healing, so self-regulation is a must. Moment-to-moment awareness, just being, allows us to connect to the mind and body. We connect to the mind through our thoughts and the body with our breathing.

What is in back of us and what is in front of us is of little importance compared to what is inside of us. What we give out comes from inside. If we have hate, anger, fear, and revenge inside us, that is what we give out. If we have love inside us, that is what we give out.

It is important to stay connected to the source, to the one, the spirit, the universal mind, God; in meditation, we come in direct contact with the one. See yourself as being the best you can be in body, mind, and spirit. You are somebody, you are loved.

CHAPTER 15
Success

Success is love, joy, and peace.
—Peter Lowe

There is no such thing as failure if you learn from it. There is no such thing as failure if you change your mind. There are no problems; you only think you have problems. If you change your mind, the problems vanish. You have control of your thoughts, and you can change them anytime you want.

Failure is an event, not a person. Tomorrow, the event may be over. According to Dr. Maxwell Maltz, success is the creative accomplishment of a goal. There are many types of goals: developmental goals include learning a language, writing a book, giving a successful speech; thing goals such as owning a car, house, or boat; and financial goals, such as investing in stocks or real estate. Finally, there are contribution goals: the more you give out, the more you get back. Be of service to others. According to Anthony Robbins, there is a success formula. Ask what you want, make a committed decision (a decision free from all other possibilities), take action, and watch what you get; you will get a result that will be good or bad. If the result is bad, keep changing until you get the desired result.

Successful action depends on your thoughts, your decisions, and your potential. The grandfather of all action is your thoughts, the father of all action is your decisions, and the master of all action is your potential. You are pure potentiality and possibility. Tap into your potentiality with empowering beliefs, empowering thoughts, and attitudes; potential energy is converted into energy of action (kinetic energy).

Actions are followed by results. The result will be good or bad, so keep changing until you get the desired result. Repetition is the mother of all learning. If you learn from something, you can't fail. In other words, there can be success even in the face of failure. Winston Churchill said that failure after failure means success. Abraham Lincoln had failure after failure and finally became president of the United States. Before Edison finally invented the electric light, he had failure after failure; he said that he learned from each failed experiment.

Success is a sense of direction, understanding, compassion, courage, self-acceptance, self-esteem, and self-confidence, while failure is frustration, aggression, misdirected aggression (like driving a car at high speed), insecurity, loneliness, uncertainty, resentment, and emptiness.

Zig Ziglar says that success is the right attitude, plus skills, plus the golden rule, plus character. Character depends on the purpose of life. The purpose of life is to be healthy and happy, and to have peace of mind, harmonious relationships at work and at home, security, reasonable prosperity, friends, and hope for a better future.

See your being full of success, doing successful activities, being successful in everything you touch, and the result is having happiness and peace of mind. Enjoy things that money can buy, and things that money cannot buy. To be successful, let others get what they want, so that you can get what you want. Success is a win-win situation.

The goal in life is to have peace of mind. See yourself as relaxed, calm, and confident. According to Dr. Wayne Dyer, there are ten rules for success and peace of mind:

Rule 1. Keep an open mind, free from all attachments. If you are not attached to anything like spouse, greed, stocks, home, real estate, or desires, you will be free.

Rule 2. Whatever you have inside of you is what you give out. If you have love inside of you, that is what you give out. If you have hate, anger, fear, or resentment, that is what you give out.

Rule 3. Play the music that you want to play. What is your purpose in life? Your archetype? For example, my primordial desire is to learn and teach. I am here to be an outstanding writer and speaker; I am here to give motivational talks. I am here to be of service to others and make a difference in this world. My values are to give love and be loved, to be healthy, to learn and teach and make a difference.

Rule 4. Embrace silence. Tap into the universal mind; come into direct contact with the one, God.

According to the Kabbalist, God is the light that shines, the light that is between our thoughts. The Kabbalist believes that we are here to receive love, happiness, peace of mind, financial security, and self-fulfillment.

It is not what is in front of us or in back of us, but what is inside of us. All the resources are inside of us in our unconscious, where the spirit, the energy, and the soul, consciousness, reside. The soul is the thinker of thoughts and creates the body/ego personality. The ego is destructive if it remains separate and disconnected from the source. There is a spiritual solution to all problems. The ego functions best if it remains connected to the source.

Rule 5. Forget about the past. Release yourself from the chains of the past and the prison of guilt. Live in the present. The thoughts of today create the future. The thoughts of today make the body of tomorrow.

Rule 6. Release yourself from resentments. Forgive yourself and others. Just as the butterfly emerges from the cocoon, love emerges from the wings of forgiveness.

Rule 7. See yourself the way you want to be, believe it, and achieve it. See yourself as loving, capable, and worthwhile. I like to see myself as an outstanding writer and speaker; believe it and achieve it. For whatever you conceive, believe you can achieve (Napoleon Hill, *Think and Grow Rich*).

Rule 8. The person who has the problem cannot solve the problem. There are no problems; you only think that you have problems. If you change your mind, you will release the problem. You have control of your thoughts; you have control of your mind. The mind has the power to heal. You can change your mind anytime you want to. Insanity is doing the same thing over and over and expecting a different result. It will never happen.

Rule 9. Cherish the divinity inside of you. You are worthy and are made in the image and likeness of God. You have God within you. In the infinity of life where I am, all is perfect, whole, and complete. All is well in my world.

Rule 10. Wisdom is releasing the lower, weaker energy, weaker frequencies, and vibrations such as anger, fear, resentment, anxiety, depression, guilt, shame, and blame and replacing them with the higher energies of love, joy, and peace. Let go of the anger and fear. You are somebody, you are love. Surrender the fear.

The Sinatra Solution

We can prevent and treat heart disease. The combination of coenzyme Q10, L-Carnitine, and D-Ribose help prevent and treat heart disease. Heart disease includes congestive heart failure (CHF), hypertension, coronary heart disease, angina, arrhythmia, and cardiomyopathy.

Congestive heart failure is a progressive disease of the heart muscle; the heart cannot function effectively as a pump. The patient is short of breath with a little exercise. There is fluid or congestion in the lungs. A chest x-ray would reveal an enlarged heart with fluid at the base. Intravenous Lasix would produce great relief. For CHF, Dr. Sinatra recommends multivitamins, coenzyme Q10 (100 mg TID), L-Carnitine (2000 mg daily), D-Ribose (15 gm), and magnesium (400 mg). Severe CHF requires an increase in the dosage of the meds if quality of life is still not satisfactory; Dr. Sinatra recommends adding 1500 mg of Hawthorne berries and 2-3 gm of Taurine.

High blood pressure is in the range of 140 to 150 over 90; high blood pressure can cause stroke, CHF, and cardiomyopathy if left untreated. Niacin (500 mg BID) lowers cholesterol, raises HDL, and lowers blood pressure. Dr. Sinatra recommends multivitamins, minerals, and fish oil: 1 gm coenzyme Q10 (150 mg BID), L-Carnitine (500 mg BD), D-Ribose (5-10 gm), magnesium (400-500 gm), fish oil (2 gm), garlic, Hawthorne berry (1000 to 1500 mg). Garlic and Hawthorne berry have similar action to angiotensin-converting enzyme (ACE) inhibitors. The Resperate unit will lower blood pressure by slowing respiration down to three breaths per minute. I recommend weight loss, salt reduction, exercise, aerobic resistance, yoga, and Pilates. Coenzyme Q10, with the help of L-Carnitine, energizes the mitochondria and increases the patient's energy levels.

Coronary artery disease is caused by a buildup of plaque in the blood vessels feeding the heart. This plaque formation restricts blood flow to the heart muscle itself and deprives the heart cells of oxygen. This is also called ischemic heart disease.

Angina pectoris is classically defined as a squeezing or pressure or even a burning-like chest pain, a "heart cramp." Angina is caused by an insufficient supply of oxygen to the heart muscle. There can be radiation of pain to the jaw or left shoulder.

The treatment for stable angina pectoris is as follows:

1. Multivitamin mineral program with 1 gm of fish oil
2. Coenzyme Q10: 100 mg twice a day
3. L-Carnitine: 2000 mg daily
4. D-Ribose: 10 to 15 gm
5. Magnesium: 400 to 800 mg

Note: I also recommend that my patients suffering from angina drink green tea every day. In one Japanese study including over five hundred men with documented coronary artery disease, a cup of green tea per day seemed to prevent a heart attack.

Cardiac arrhythmia is an irregular heartbeat, characterized by an increased or decreased heart rate or a "skipped" heartbeat, also called heart palpitation. The treatment for arrhythmia is magnesium, coenzyme Q10, L-Carnitine, D-Ribose, and alpha-linolenic acid. Omega 3 (in fish) helps cardiovascular health.

High blood pressure can cause strokes and kidney failure. Diet and lifestyle play a big part in the management of hypertension. There is no reason for you to have high blood pressure. High blood pressure is a man-made disease.

Let me list the things you can do to lower and control your blood pressure:

1. CoQ10, L-Carnitine, and D-Ribose.
2. Resperate: a device that lowers blood pressure by slowing down your breathing (ideally three breaths per minute).
3. Lose weight and cut down on salt. Salt increases your fluid volume.
4. All diseases benefit from exercise. Exercise for thirty minutes, five times per week.
5. A healthy Mediterranean diet: Five veggies and three fruits, legumes, grains and nuts, garlic, eight to ten glasses of clean water, cold-water fish (mackerel, sardines, herring, cod, halibut),

cruciferous veggies (cabbage, broccoli, Brussels sprouts, spinach, kale, and cauliflower). Consider clean air, organic food, and clean water free from lead, mercury, and cadmium. Follow the nutrition guidelines for hypertension.

6. Reduce stress: stress (physical and mental) stimulates the sympathetic nervous system, resulting in increased BP and heart rate. Transcendental meditation, self-hypnosis, and Hatha yoga lower blood pressure.

7. Learn to check your blood pressure at home, use relaxation techniques, and observe the lowering of blood pressure. Check your blood pressure before and after meditation.

8. Stop smoking, alcohol, caffeine, and concentrated sugar.

9. Add 40 gm of soluble fiber to your diet.

10. Add calcium, magnesium, and potassium to your diet in the form of supplements; 1000 mg of calcium and magnesium are a must. Calcium lowers blood pressure, and magnesium stops arrhythmias and prevents coronary spasm.

CHAPTER 16
Who Am I?

I spent many years trying to determine who I really am. Early in my life, I was very dependent and needed much support. I felt unworthy and incompetent, searching for meaning in all this suffering. I constantly heard my mother's voice: "Watch what you say." I was apprehensive and suffered from social anxiety. I felt uncomfortable getting in front of an audience and giving a speech. I had low self-esteem and a poor self-image. I felt abandoned as a child, as my parents spent most of their time operating a grocery store. They gave their time to the customers. My parents cared for me in their own way; they never said that they loved me. My dad never received any love from his parents. He was abused as a child. I cannot fault him. I now can respect and love him.

My self-esteem improved in high school; I graduated third in a class of 365, and I graduated from medical school in the top of my class. Now I feel worthy and competent. I see myself as capable, loving, and worthwhile. I regard myself as an outstanding writer and speaker. I am a gentle listener, and I enjoy learning and teaching.

I am more patient and stay connected to my source. I respect myself and others, supported by thoughts, words, and actions. I am the best I can be in everything I do. I am the best physically, mentally, and spiritually. I attempt to be in an imagined state of perfection. I am an idealist. I feel connected to people and enjoy being with people, particularly positive and interesting people.

Life is impermanent and is constantly changing; we can change and grow. It is helpful to have a partner who is your friend and helps you on the way. My wife has been that partner, and I don't think that I would have overcome all the negatives that I had without her help. Virginia helped me get over my social anxiety and keep changing until I got the desired result.

A mind that creates a problem cannot solve it. We need help. We must change our thinking, change our mind, in order to solve problems. If we keep doing the same thing, we get the same results. The important lesson is that we have total control of our mind; we have the choice to change our minds at any time.

We ask what we want and make a committed decision, followed by action and a result. The result can be good or bad; if the result is disastrous, keep changing until you get a desired result. This formula makes for success. Remember that failure is an event, not a person. And there is no such thing as failure if we learn from it.

Winston Churchill said that success is one failure after another. Churchill failed English three times and went on to become a great orator. Abe Lincoln held only one state office before becoming president.

We are all here on this planet for a purpose. My purpose is to learn and teach. I also want harmonious relationships and have friends and hope for a better future (of course, financial security is included).

The main problem in Western society is we think that we are not good enough, unworthy. We must learn to love ourselves.

I learned the following mirror exercise from Louise Hay:

Look in the mirror each morning and say, "I love myself, therefore I feel better. I love myself, therefore I can think, feel, and behave better. I love myself, therefore I take care of my body, my home, my spouse, my children. I am loving, capable, and worthwhile. If I have love inside of me, that is what I give out. If I have hate inside of me, that is what I give out. If I give service to others, I am rewarded manyfold."

Anxiety causes stress and a release of adrenalin, due to the stimulation of the sympathetic nervous system. There is rapid irregular breathing, a rapid heart rate, an increase in BP, blood clots, an increase in blood sugar, and increased muscle tension. Hypnosis and meditation slow the breathing and make it regular. The heart rate and blood pressure come down; the anxious person may have palpitations, hyperventilation, queasy stomach, headache, and so on. Learn to breathe through your nose and count from 5 to 1; with each count, become more and more relaxed. Use deep relaxation and visual imagery. See yourself confronting the situation with success, confidence, and the winning way. I leave you with my favorite poem:

Every moment of love,
Every moment of giving,
Every moment of joy,
Is a moment of living.
Every moment of anger,
Every moment of lying,
Every moment of fear,
Is a moment of dying.

Place your thumbs and index fingers together, take three deep breaths, and say, "I am relaxed, calm, and confident." See yourself as relaxed, calm, and confident. Believe it and achieve it. Whatever you conceive, believe you can achieve. Positive mental images make you feel good and behave better, just as positive self-talk activates neurotransmitters like endorphins, dopamine, norepinephrine, and serotonin (feel good hormone).

Place your thumb and index finger together, forming a zero. Now, count down from 5 to 1; with each count, feel more and more relaxed. Milton Erickson deepens the trance by using the hand levitation exercise or the reverse levitation. The hand becomes very light and automatically floats up to the face, and when it touches the face, you will become twice as relaxed. One can also add numbness for analgesia.

Picture the sun on the beach at dawn. Behind the clouds watch the sun change colors from orange, red, golden yellow to white. Feel the warmth of the sun, smell the fresh air, hear the sound of the waves, and watch the waves as they go in and out and you become more and more relaxed. Taste the salt water. You are now relaxed, calm, and confident. You can use any positive reference memory that will make you feel good and behave better.

My favorite inductions are eye fixation, breathing exercises, count down from 5 to 1, somnambulism (amnesia and dissociation), Esdaile's coma, hand levitation, and reverse levitation. Hand levitation allows the hands to become numb and transfers the numbness to other parts of the body: abdomen, back, and jaw (for dental anesthesia).

In my practice (thirty-five years' experience), I have used hypnosis for the following:

1. Smoking cessation
2. Weight reduction
3. Insomnia
4. Anxiety, depression, phobias
5. Irritable bowel syndrome
6. Asthma
7. Back and neck pain, bursitis
8. Alcohol addiction
9. Migraine and tension headaches
10. Hypertension
11. Cancer
12. Impotence and frigidity
13. Child birth
14. Stress management

CHAPTER 17
Aloe Vera

A colleague asked me about the benefits of aloe vera. Here is what I told her:

The benefits of pure aloe vera are well known. Aloe has been used for thousands of years for many ailments. The vitamins, minerals, and enzymes in this plant allow your immune system to function at its best. Aloe can be made into a nutritional drink that stimulates the birth of new healthy tissue.

My favorite aloe juice is New Vitality 18X, which has eighteen times more mucopolysaccharide than ordinary aloe juice. Aloe works from the inside out in moisturizing the skin. It is the mucopolysaccharides in the aloe that moisturize the skin.

You can mix aloe juice with your favorite beverage. In the morning, I add a half ounce of aloe juice to eight ounces of apple or orange juice, or water. You can also mix the aloe with half apple juice and orange juice. You can make a smoothie by adding a banana and put it in a blender. Initially, I would suggest that you use one ounce of the aloe vera juice and then cut it to a half ounce. I have a juicer, Juiceman 11, and I make my own fruit and vegetable juices and add the aloe to them. I also add Superfood Greens Plus, with grasses, probiotics, and standardized herbal and botanical extracts: three teaspoonfuls to eight ounces of juice.

Aloe vera also speeds up wound healing. A study in the *Journal of the American Podiatric Medical Association* found that aloe preparations improved wound healing. Another study in the *Journal of Alternative Medicine* found that aloe vera juice can be effective for treating inflammatory bowel disease and improving bowel regularity. Aloe contains at least three anti-inflammatory fatty acids, and this explains why aloe vera is such an effective treatment for burns, cuts, and abrasions. All these benefits occur by taking aloe internally.

I have been taking aloe juice internally for many years and have noticed tremendous improvement in my skin. I am eighty years of age and my skin remains free of wrinkles.

CHAPTER 18
Alzheimer's Disease

Alzheimer's disease is caused by chronic stress and the stress hormone cortisol. The brain can be regenerated; there are four elements that can help: nutrition, stress management, exercise, and pharmacology (ginkgo biloba and phosphatidylserine). Life Extension's Gingoathere is an inverse relationship between cortisol and DHEA. The higher the DHEA, the lower the cortisol. DHEA can help patients with Alzheimer's. Conventional doctors prescribe the choline-esterase inhibitors, Aricept and Exelon. These agents do not stop the progression of the disease. Life Extension recommends Curcumin (Turmeric) and Ashwaganda. These agents will stop the progression of the disease. The recommended protocol is exercise, Greens Plus with 18X Aloe Vera, DHEA, gingko biloba, and phosphatidylserine (100 mg TID). The dose of ginkgo is 240 mg daily.

If severe stress continues, the result is chronic high levels of cortisol with memory loss and overall cognitive decline. L-Depenyl (5 mg) will enhance memory and increase dopamine (this stops abnormal movement). I would be remiss not to mention the classic *Brain Longevity* by Dharma Singh Khalsa, MD. The brain is electrical and needs stimulation. Cranial electrotherapy stimulation results in euphoric relaxation and takes care of depression and insomnia. The alpha stimulation of the brain requires electrodes to the ears and 9 volt stimulation for twenty minutes; I personally do twenty minutes of cranial electrotherapy stimulation on a daily basis.

Anti-aging medicine is the future of medicine. Bio-identical hormone replacement is an important component of anti-aging medicine. The anti-aging doctor looks for the cause of the problem, while the conventional doctor looks for the disease. Conventional medicine is disease oriented. Initially, blood testing is done. The anti-aging doctor tests for adrenal hormones, DHEA, and cortisol, the stress hormone.

He also checks for the sex hormones estrogen (estradiol), progesterone, and testosterone. Prostate disease is age related; if you live to by age eighty-five, you have a 45 percent chance of having prostate cancer. If it is a localized form of prostate cancer and it is of no consequence, you don't die of the disease. You die with the prostate still in you.

Conventional doctors also check for thyroid and insulin growth factor, IGFI. After the hormones are balanced and there is a deficiency of IGFI, then consider the injections of the growth hormone. I am age eighty-eight and had a low level of testosterone. My anti-aging doctor recommended hormone replacement with 100 mg of testosterone cream (not the injection). I use the cream transdermally on my inner thighs every morning.

My testosterone level is now normal and my estradiol is normal. There is a hormonal balance between my estradiol and testosterone. My vitamin D3 is low, and my doctor recommended 5000 vitamin D units BID.

We age because of decreasing hormones, free radical damage, and environmental pollution. The anti-aging doctor looks for the cause and prevention of the problem to strengthen my prostate. If you have a deficiency of IGFI, ask your doctor about the Trans-D Tropic Protocols to mimic and release growth hormone. There are three ways to lower estradiol: zinc (50 mg), Super Miraforte, and Anastrazole (1 mg weekly).

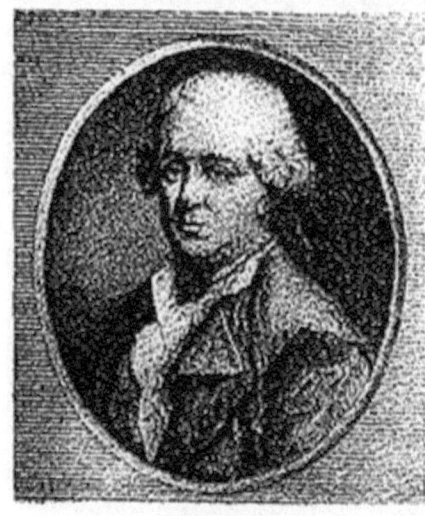

Franz Anton Mesmer
1734-1815

Mesmer was a German Physician, and was considered the Inventor of animal magnetism.

He first distinguished himself by publishing a thesis while in the University of Vienna in 1766 "Dissertation upon the Influence of the Stars on the Human Body."

He was so successful in Paris with mesmerism that the number of patients increased so rapidly and his cures were so numerous and exciting that he organised a number of pupils to administer animal magnetism under his supervision.

In 1779 he published a dissertation on the "Discovery of Animal Magnetism."

Struck with the clearness and accuracy of his reasonings, the extraordinary and unquestionable cures he performed, that some of the greatest and most prominent physicians, philosophers of France became his converts.

While Mesmer's success was short-lived, his technique was picked up and used in both England and the United States.

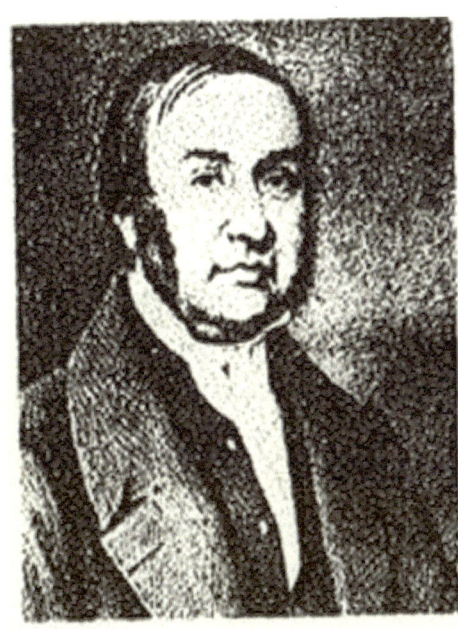

James Braid
1795-1860

Braid was an English surgeon who studied hypnosis
intifically. He played an important part in rescuing that
ince from ignorance and supersitition. It was he who
ied the word "hypnosis" from the Greek word hypnos,
ining sleep.

"My chief objective is not to exploit those elements
: give rise to supersititious and magical belief, but to
ure that everything mystical is excluded from the circle
scientific hypnotic practice."

J. Braid, 1842

"Hypnotism cannot but arouse the special interest of all
:tising doctors, theoreticians, lawyers, ministers and in-
d every man who would perfect and validate his know-
ie of human nature."

J. Braid, 1842

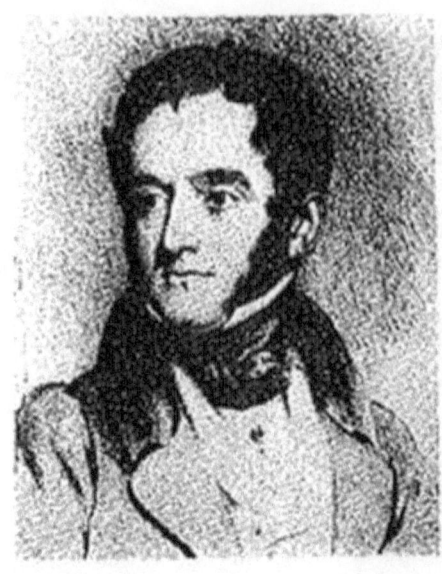

John Elliotson
1791-1862

Elliotson was the great chest specialist who brought the stethoscope to England.

He was the first Professor of Medicine at the newly established University of London.

He was the leader of the Mesmeric Movement in London. He began to treat patients with mesmerism and gave lectures and demonstrations which attracted large and distinguished audiences. He was severely criticized by his colleagues and urged to desist by the Dean by the School, and was called a professional pariah by the Lancet. Undaunted Elliotson carried on his work in mesmerism, started a journal called the Zoist in 1842 for the express purpose of propagating mesmerism. The thirteen volumes continued up till 1856 and provided a wealth of information in all branches of mesmeric sciences.

On June 27, 1848, he delivered the Harveian Oration before the Royal College of Physicians in London, and mesmerism was the subject of his address.

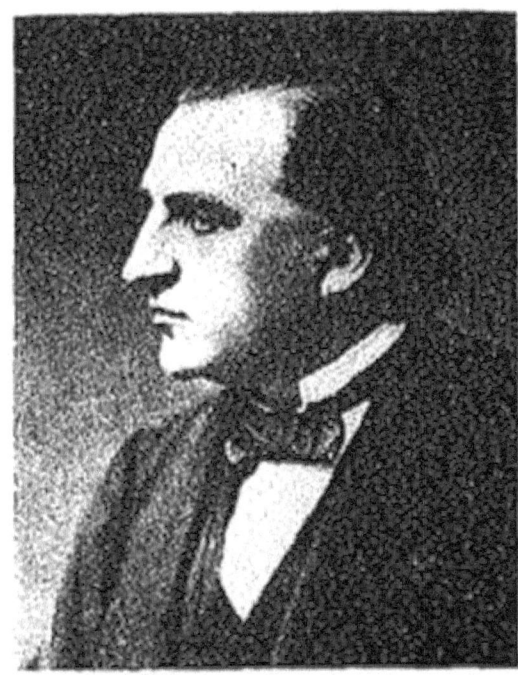

Jean Martin
Charcot
1825-1893

Charcot was the most distinguished neurologist of the
th Century. He was the founder of the Paris School of
pnosis.

He developed an interest in hypnosis, and began his
blic classes at the School of Salpetiere in which he
ected attention to the physical states of hystero-epileptics
ring hypnosis. Charcot thought that hypnosis and hysteria
ıre identical.

Charcot's interest in hypnosis made the subject respect-
le and was followed by a large number of medical men
Europe.

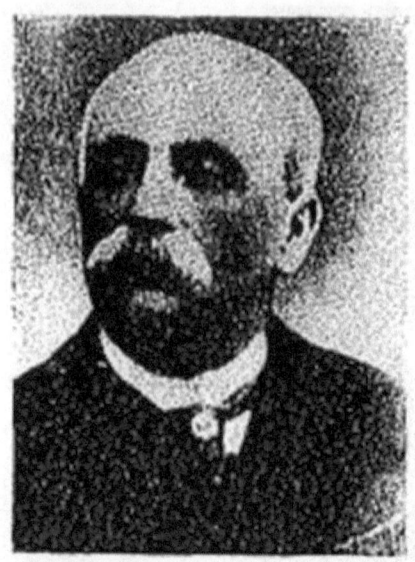

Hippolyte-Marie Bernheim
1840-1919

Bernheim was a famous physician, and was a professor of clinical medicine at Nancy.

It was Bernheim who stripped the subject of hypnosis of much of its mystery, dispelled ideas of special hypnotic powers and magnetic influences, and demonstrated that patients were also susceptible to suggestion in the walking state.

At the beginning Bernheim was sceptical and incredulous about hypnosis. In France during that time Dr. Liebeault was treating thousands of patients suffering from a great assortment of physical symptoms; and in 1882 he cured an obstinate case of sciatica, of six years' duration, which Bernheim had treated in vain for six months. Incensed by the claims of Liebeault, Bernheim decided to visit his clinic to expose him as a quack. He was instead so amazed at Liebeault's work that he undertook a study of hypnotism, and he soon became one of its most ardent devotees. He led the School of Nancy and developed a psychological approach to the theory of hypnosis based on the influence of suggestion, and opposed to the Paris Hospital of Salpetriere led by Charcot who believed that hypnosis was a pathogical phenomenon akin to hysteria, the product of an abnormal nervous constitution.

Bernheim wrote a book De La Suggestion et de Ses Applications a La Therapeutique in 1884.

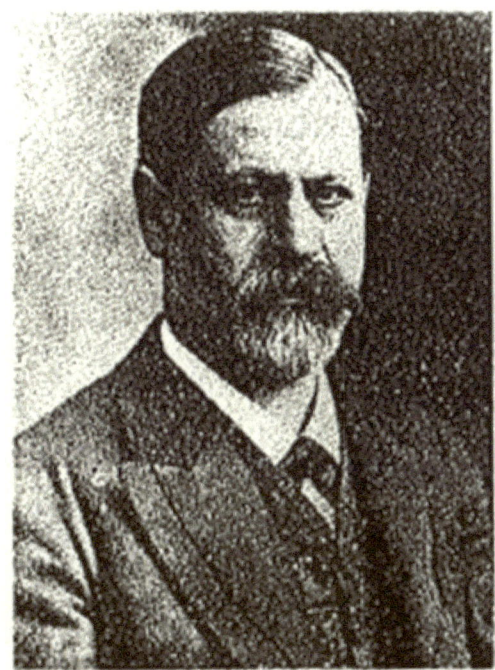

Sigmund Freud
1856-1939

Sigmund Freud became acquainted with hypnosis when saw a stage performance by the famous lay hypnotist nsen. At first he questioned the genuineness of the ɛnomena, but he was convinced by the paleness of a ɔject when cataleptic rigidity was produced.

Later Freud studied hypnosis under Charcot and rnheim.

Freud finally abandoned hypnosis because "not all sub- ts can develop a deep trance", and that "the removal of nptoms by hypnosis was often temporary and that the nptoms would either return or be replaced by others".

Freud's rejection of hypnosis was a great blow to the ɪ of hypnosis in psychotherapy because his followers ːepted his teachings as unalterable dogma.

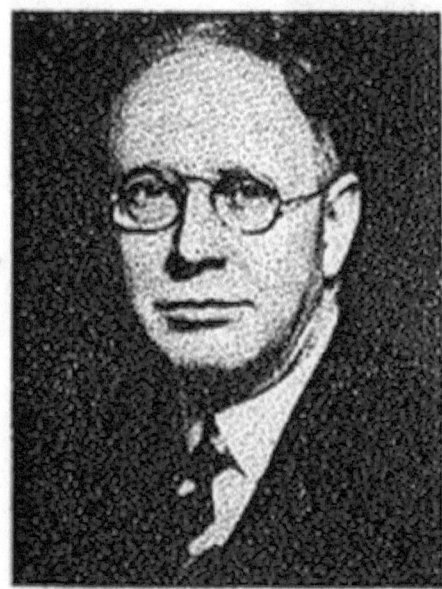

Clark L. Hull
1884-1952

    C. L. Hull, one of the great leaders in the exploration of learning theory, was one of the pioneers whose outstanding work in the direction of bringing hypnosis out of the field of clinical and abnormal psychology and subjecting it to more rigorous scientific experimentation. In his book, Hypnosis and Suggestibility Hull summarises the process of thinking, and points to a number of experiments which demonstrate "a remarkable and detailed conformity of the phenomena of hypnosis to the known experimental characteristics of ordinary habituations".

re Janet 1859-1947

Janet was attracted to the Salpetriere in Paris by the
·k of Charcot on Hysteria and Hypnotism.

He became Professor of Psychology in the College de
ice.   He studied particularly the various phenomena of
gestion, phobias, automatism and compulsive acts and
ught together in one systematic framework all the strange
nomena of hysteria.

Janet introduced the concepts of dissociation of psycho-
cal tension, and that of a subconscious.

He played an important part in the discovery of some
the essential tenets of modern psychology and laid the
undwork for an explanative psychopathology.   His con-
utions as a pioneer in psychological medicine merit much
itude.

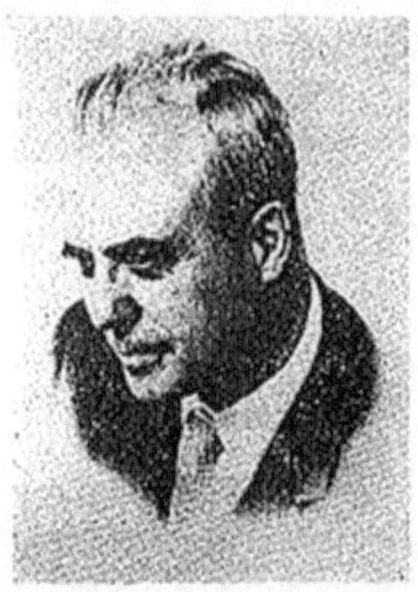

Milton H. Erickson
Born Dec. 5, 1901

Milton H. Erickson, M.D. is a leading exponent of hypnotic techniques and research in the United States. He received his early training at the University of Winsconsin and was certified by the American Board of Psychiatry and Neurology in 1939.

He was formerly Chief Psychiatrist, Research Service, Worcester State Hospital, Worcester, Massachusetts, 1930-1934; Director of Psychiatric Research, 1934-1939, Wayne County General Hospital, Eloise, Michigan. He was later Director of Research and Psychiatric Training, 1939-1948 at the same institution.

Among his numerous previous teaching posts, he was an Instructor in Psychiatry, 1939-1940; Assistant Professor and Associate Professor of Psychiatry, 1940-1948, at Wayne State University College of Medicine Detroit, Michigan. He served as Senior Member, Teaching Faculty, Seminars on Hypnosis, Chicago, Illinois, 1955-1961.

It was during the 1930's, when new research in hypnosis was evolving, that Dr. Erickson was the first to investigate the effects of hypnosis on psychological and physiological behaviour. The work as laid down by Erickson was later followed in experimental studies by Clark L. Hull, a research psychologist at Yale, while the author pursued his own studies of hypnosis in psychiatry.

CHAPTER 19

Secrets of Hypnosis

The word "hypnosis" was coined by James Braid in 1840. He thought that hypnosis was a form of sleep. This is incorrect, because someone in a trance state is alert. Through the years, there have been many definitions for hypnosis. In the eighteenth century, Anton Mesmer thought that it was caused by magnetism.

Goullitine and Benjamin Franklin investigated Mesmer and called him a fraud. They thought that mesmerism was due to imagination. In the early 1900s, Bernheim and Liebault thought that hypnosis was a state of hypersuggestibility. Bernheim wrote a book on his findings called *Hypnosis and Suggestion.*

In Paris, Dr. Charcot, a neurologist, viewed hypnosis as a form of hysteria and treated hysterical cases, such as hysterical paralysis, with hypnosis. Sigmund Freud studied under Bernheim and Charcot. Sigmund Freud was not a good hypnotist and abandoned hypnosis for free association and psychoanalysis.

James Esdaile, a Scottish surgeon, went to India and performed three hundred operations using hypnosis instead of anesthesia. He developed a form of somnambulism, Esdaile's coma. His procedures took two hours to produce a deep enough trance to do surgery. Many of his operations were for scrotal tumors and amputation. Dr. Ainsle Mears of Melbourne, Australia, thought that hypnosis was due to atavism—a regression to a primitive, caveman existence where suggestion and not critical judgment played a part in everyday existence. The brain and its prefrontal area were not developed enough to be judgmental, and to analyze and compare. According to Dr. Milton Erickson, the father of modern hypnosis, hypnosis is an altered state of consciousness, a communication of ideas to the unconscious, which accepts them unequivocally and carries them out. The unconscious has all the resources you need.

R. Morris defines hypnosis as a state of mind, whereby one has mental control, emotional control, and attitudinal control. I define hypnosis as a state of mind, a mood whereby one bypasses critical judgment and replaces it with selective thinking and selective awareness. Hypnosis requires both physical and mental relaxation.

See yourself as relaxed, calm, and confident; believe it and achieve it. Whatever you conceive, believe you can achieve. Positive mental images make you feel good and behave better, just as positive self-talk activates neurotransmitters like endorphins, dopamine, norepinephrine, and serotonin (feel-good hormone).

Place your thumb and index finger together, forming a zero. Now, count down from 5 to 1, with each count feel more and more relaxed. Milton Erickson deepens the trance by using the hand levitation exercise or the reverse levitation. The hand becomes very light and automatically floats up to the face, and when it touches the face, you will become twice as relaxed. One can also add numbness for analgesia.

Picture the sun on the beach at dawn. Behind the clouds, watch the sun change colors from orange, red, golden yellow to white. Feel the warmth of the sun, smell the fresh air, hear the sound of the waves, and watch the waves as they go in and out, and you become more and more relaxed. Taste the salt water. You are now relaxed, calm, and confident. You can use any positive reference memory that will make you feel good and behave better.

My favorite inductions are eye fixation, breathing exercises, count down from 5 to 1, somnambulism (amnesia and dissociation), Esdaile's coma, hand levitation, and reverse levitation. Milton Erickson deepens relaxation with the hand levitation: allow the hands to become numb, and transfer the numbness to other parts of the body: abdomen, back, and jaw (for dental anesthesia).

In my practice (thirty-five years' experience), I have used hypnosis for the following:

1. Smoking cessation
2. Weight reduction
3. Insomnia
4. Anxiety, depression, phobias
5. Irritable bowel syndrome

6. Asthma
7. Back and neck pain, bursitis
8. Alcohol addiction
9. Migraine and tension headaches
10. Hypertension
11. Cancer
12. Impotence and frigidity
13. Child birth
14. Stress management
15. Gynecological conditions

High blood pressure is a man-made disease and can be prevented. There is no reason for anyone to suffer from heart disease. Blood pressure readings are systole divided by diastole. The normal pressure is around 120 over 80. The numerator (or systole) means contraction of the heart and the denominator (or diastole) is the relaxation.

High blood pressure can cause a heart attack, stroke, or congestive heart failure. A good metaphor for normal blood pressure is a table top supported by four legs:

1. A healthy Mediterranean diet and lifestyle
2. Nutritional supplements and herbs
3. Exercise
4. Stress management: self-hypnosis, meditation, yoga, and anger management

The hypertensive patient needs calcium, magnesium, and potassium. They have a deficiency of these minerals and must focus on foods in the diet that can supply them:

Cabbage, broccoli, kale, and cauliflower supply calcium and potassium as well as folic acid and vitamin E. Calcium and potassium can help lower BP. Folic acid can protect the heart and, along with B12, can lower homocysteine. High homocysteine can cause a heart attack, even if all the lipids and other risk factors are normal. Remember that cabbage has Indole 3 Carbinol, which can protect against breast cancer. Cabbage juice can cure ulcers. Magnesium, potassium, and fiber are found in legumes. Beans such as lentils, chickpeas, red kidney beans, and cannelloni are high in fiber, low in fat, and rich in protein;

they contain a good supply of magnesium and potassium, which are wonderful for lowering your blood pressure. Magnesium can prevent heart irregularities and spasm of the coronary arteries.

Fiber lowers cholesterol and slows the absorption of carbs. The soy bean contains magnesium and omega 3, alpha-linolenic acid. Omega 3 can protect against heart disease. The soy-based foods are tofu, tempeh, and miso. Today, one can purchase soy cheese and meats, including soy hot dogs and veggie burgers.

Cold-water fish—salmon, mackerel, sardines, and herring—contain omega 3s and coenzyme Q10. Salmon twice a week can cut sudden death by 50 percent. CoQ10 strengthens the heart muscle and increases cellular energy; it acts as a spark for the mitochondria in the heart and aids the oxidation of fat.

I had the pleasure of meeting and working with Dr. Jon Kabot Zinn, author of *Mindfulness Meditation*. He posed a question to me: What is the difference between hypnosis and meditation? In hypnosis, we bypass the critical judgment and replace it with selective thinking, like stress reduction or freedom from pain.

In meditation there is non-doing, just being. Now, I am a silent witness to nothing and the sacred space between thoughts, where there is God, universal mind, imagination, creativity, and cosmic consciousness as a silent witness. I can observe the mind in action, the incessant thoughts. I am not my thoughts; my goal is to free myself from thoughts. Let my thoughts go. Mindfulness meditation reduces stress. Mindfulness meditation is nonjudgmental, moment-to-moment awareness; as long as I breathe through my nose, there are no thoughts. There is power in thoughts; thoughts create reality and the future, but there is more power in no thoughts. No thoughts are deeply relaxing and reduce stress. Hypnosis requires thinking and doing, while meditation requires non-doing, just being. My being is still and peaceful.

CHAPTER 20

Self-Talk

Positive self-talk is a conversation with the self. Positive self-talk enhances performance and self-image. Positive self-talk activates the brain and releases the neurotransmitters endorphins, dopamine, norepinephrine, and serotonin (the feel-good hormone).

I, Anthony, am honest and have integrity, I am optimistic and enthusiastic, I am goal-directed and goal-oriented. I am punctual. I am responsible for my actions without blaming. My power stays with me. I am committed; I am energetic and active; I am organized and detail-oriented. I am orderly and free from clutter; I like a nice-looking, clean office.

I am motivated. I am love. I am the best I can be every day. I love myself, God, and my neighbor. I look in the mirror and say, "Anthony, I love you; therefore, I can think, feel, and behave better."

I am loving, capable, and worthwhile. I am worthy. I am changeable and release myself from my comfort zone. I am growing and changing. I am healthy and happy. I think pleasant thoughts most of the time. I am teachable and I am a gentle listener. I listen and then am understood. I am happy with my relationships at home and at work. I am reasonably prosperous and secure. I am pleased with my friends, and I hope for a bright future. There are bigger and brighter days ahead.

I am committed. I am respectful of myself and others, supported by thoughts, words, and actions. I release negative thoughts and feelings and attract loving thoughts. I am patient and am connected to the source. I am full of loving kindness and give loving kindness to others. I am whole, healthy, strong, and vital. I am opulent and abundant. I am an outstanding writer and speaker. Believe it and achieve it.

I see myself as I want to be. I am already the way I want to be. I want to be happy and healthy, be reasonably prosperous, have peace of mind, and have secure harmonious relationships at home and at work, an abundance of friends, and hope for a bright future. I am a difference maker, locally and globally.

I am learning and teaching, and I feel good. I am a service to mankind. I am playing the music I have inside of me, and I am releasing the love I have inside of me. I am determined and persistent. I am patient. I am creative and imaginative. I have an open mind and am free to do what I want to do. I am pure potentiality and consciousness, I am successful, I creatively move toward my goal, my target. I be before I do, and I do before I have. I am relaxed, calm, and confident. I am the ideal self. The best.

CHAPTER 21
The Power of Thoughts

The universe is made of energy and motion. Beneath all solids are atoms, molecules moving at lightning speed. The solids are made of electrons, neutrons, protons, and subatomic particles. Thoughts are everywhere. The mind is in every cell of our bodies. The mind is in every immune cell. Each cell talks to each other chemically. The cells communicate by means of neuropeptides.

Thoughts are energy and can be afflictive or healthy. The healthy thoughts are love, joy, and peace. In fact, happiness is thinking pleasant thoughts most of the time, while unpleasant thoughts make us feel unhappy. When we are depressed, angry, sad, and fearful, we feel down.

The amazing thing is that we can change thoughts. We can change our minds. If our thoughts are down, we change them so that they are upbeat. Don't allow negative thoughts to enter your mind. When you experience a negative thought, say, "Stop!" You can even snap a rubber band on your wrist to stop unpleasant thoughts.

Where do these thoughts come from? They come from the light in the space between thoughts. The space between thoughts is where we have insight, imagination, and creativity. The light is God, unconditional love, the universal mind. The universal mind is like a dynamo, where all the power comes from. I believe that the gap between thoughts is the higher consciousness, the higher frequency, and vibrations of the cosmic consciousness. The cosmic consciousness allows us to be one with God and is a loving, healing tunnel to infinity and the beginning of time. In other words, we have within us all the resources we need; we have the wisdom of Socrates, Aristotle, Machiavelli, Buddha, Jesus, Leonardo da Vinci, Michelangelo, Freud, Jung, Einstein, Newton. We are pure consciousness, and with empowering beliefs and the right attitude, we can increase our potential, take action, and get results. The ancestor of all action is our thoughts, while the father of all action is our decisions. It is the moment of decision that shapes our destiny. After we make a committed decision, take action and a result will follow. It may be good or bad, but we can always change it. There are many levels of consciousness (ego consciousness, objective consciousness, individual consciousness, subjective consciousness, spirit, and soul). The spirit is the source and is energy, while the soul is pure awareness. The key is to stay connected to the source, the spirit, God. It is the ego, with its hatred, anger, fear, despair, doubt, injuries, resentment, violence, and rage, that causes the problems in society. It is a lack of spirituality. The paradox is the spirit needs the ego.

The ego needs the spirit. We must be connected to the source, the spirit, the energy of life. The self is impermanent and moves from self to no-self. When we embrace silence by meditation, we connect to the spirit and leave the ego behind. The ego is the cause of all our problems. We are constantly moving from ego-consciousness to the subconscious. The subconscious is automatic, spontaneous, and creative, and it is where all the action takes place. The willpower, the objective consciousness, the ego is analytical and does not do anything; the inner self is where all the action is. So, it is necessary to communicate with the unconscious to get things done. The unconscious has all the resources from the beginning of time. Milton Erickson was of the opinion that all the resources we need are in the unconscious. Life is a double thread: the ego and the spirit.

In the Western world, we have a problem with self-esteem. The biggest problem is feeling unworthy. This opinion is voiced by Louise Hay. We strive to be loving, capable, and worthwhile. According to Napoleon Hill in *Think and Grow Rich*, whatever we create and believe, we can achieve. He believes that if we have a burning desire, a thought, a picture that we create in our imagination, the idea, enhanced by faith, will be manifested as a thought form. In other words, everything in our environment was first present in someone's mind. Look around you; the television, the computer, the chairs, the wheel were first an idea in someone's mind. When there is a conflict between the imagination and the willpower, imagination will always win. Whatever we picture, imagine, believe, we can achieve. If I picture myself as an outstanding writer, focus on it on a daily basis, and believe it, I can achieve it. If I picture myself as an outstanding speaker and believe it, I can achieve it.

It is also wise to picture yourself and tell your universal mind that you are whole, healthy, strong, and vital; if you believe it, you can achieve it. Creative imagination is a powerful tool. Shakti Gawain wrote a fascinating book on creative imagination.

The Buddhists don't have a problem with the ego and self-esteem. They are introverted and focus their attention on the no-self and meditation. They leave the ego and bypass the critical judgment and replace it with moment-to-moment awareness. In the silence of the mind, they are a silent witness and observe the thoughts, feelings, images, sensations, and sounds, and they don't do anything. The mind connects to the body automatically through the breathing. The thoughts are incessant and never stop as the sensory input passes by; just go back to the breathing. In meditation, you don't attempt to accomplish anything, just observe.

Every thought has a feeling; in the shadow of every thought is a feeling. We have afflictive and healthy emotions. The healthy feelings—love, joy, and peace—make us feel good, while the unhealthy feelings—depression, anger, sadness, fear, hatred, ignorance, jealousy, and arrogance—make us feel unhappy. When we think of a Monet painting such as *The Japanese Bridge* or *Water Lilies,* we feel vibrant and up, but when we think of Dachau and the Holocaust, we feel sad and down. So there is a definite relationship between our thoughts and feelings. I refer you to *Emotional Intelligence* by Dr. Daniel Coleman for a detailed description of our emotions.

Did you ever think of how we get depressed? Depression is based on the way we hold our body and the state we are in. Put your shoulders and head down, move slowly, and don't smile. This puts you in a depressed state. If you hold your head up high, keep your shoulders up, move swiftly, and smile, it puts you in an upbeat state and takes you out of the depression.

Everything starts with a burning desire and a thought. A thought is energy and is enhanced by faith. Where there is doubt, let there be faith. If we take the thought and add a dose of creative imagination, we can transform an idea, a concept, into a thought form.

The mind has the power to heal. The mind can heal the body and overcome illness. There is a mind-body connection, and it is supported by scientific evidence. In psychoneuroimmunology, the mind influences the nervous system and the immune system. When we have fear, performance suffers, and there is a weakening of the immune system, a drop in the natural killer cells. This makes us vulnerable to disease.

The foundation of all healing is love. Love conquers fear. Healing depends on a healthy attitude and positive self-talk. This leads to psychological and physiological balance and wholeness instead of conflict. According to the World Health Organization, health is a state of body, mind, heart, and spiritual well-being. There is an inverse relationship between wellness and illness. The higher the state of wellness, the lower the illness. Wellness depends on a healthy Mediterranean diet: fruits, veggies, beans, grains and nuts, nutritional supplements, vitamins, coenzyme Q10, and alpha lipoic acid. If you exercise (one mile of brisk walking in fifteen minutes), you will improve the mind-body connection. Meditation, self-hypnosis, and yoga also help.

According to the Eastern philosophy, clinging to self, staying attached to self, causes sickness.

CHAPTER 22

On Becoming Eighty

On Becoming Eighty
By Frank

Today, dear Lord, I am 80,
But there's so such I haven't done.
Dear Lord, please let me live,
Until I am 81.

But wait, dear Lord, I am not through,
Permit me to ask of you,
Would you please let me stay,
until I'm 82?

So many places I'd like to be,
And so much for me to see;
so you think you could manage,
To make it 83?

There's many things I haven't done,
So much left in store,
So, I ask you, Lord,
If I may live,
until I'm 84?

But if by then, I'm still alive,
I'll kneel and take the risk,
That you'll be mad, dear Lord,
If I ask for 86?

I know, it's a lot to ask,
and know it would be nice in heaven,
but can you let me hang around,
until I'm 87?

I know by then I won't be fast,
And at times, I would be late,
But it would be, oh so great,
To be 'round, til I'm 88.

I will have seen so many things,
And have had a wonderful time,
So I'm sure I'd be so willing,
To stay to 89, uh, "Or more—maybe."

CHAPTER 23

Prostate Cancer

My urologist, Dr. Tocci, said after my rectal exam that my prostate was irregular and that I had localized prostatic cancer, but at age eighty-eight, it is of no concern. Oncologist Dr. Jeremy Geffen said that prostate cancer is age related; by eighty-eight, 43 percent have prostate cancer.

Dr. Wood, my oncologist at Life Extension, is of the opinion that localized prostate cancer can spread and one must do everything possible to prevent the spreading. Dr. Wood recommended the following:

1- One pomegranate extract capsule daily
2- Two ultra saw palmetto capsules daily
3- Vitamin D3 hormone: 5000 TU BID
4- Indole 3 Carbinol caps: 200 mg BID
5- A cruciferous diet: cabbage, broccoli, kale, cauliflower
6- Progesterone cream applied at bedtime (rub the cream into the thigh or inner arms)

Dr. Wood thinks this treatment is controversial. Dr. Philip Lee Miller of Life Extension Revolution recommends progesterone cream for prostate cancer. Progesterone cream is very relaxing and promotes sleep. I think that Dr. Wood's program makes sense and is ideal for someone with localized prostate cancer.

CHAPTER 24

Breast Cancer

If I had breast cancer, my goal would be to enhance my immune system, lymphocytes, macrophages, and natural killer cells and learn how to handle stress. Conventional treatments for cancer have made little progress through the years: Surgery, radiation, and chemotherapy have done little to improve the cancer situation. We need to look for alternative effective, nontoxic therapies. According to Charles B. Simone, MD, author of *Cancer Nutrition*, 90 percent of all cancers are related to nutritional factors. Diet and lifestyle are paramount; we need five vegetables and three fruits on a daily basis. Our lifestyle should center on avoiding tobacco, smoking, excessive alcohol, high animal fat, high cholesterol, and environmental pollution.

The best way to get the veggies and fruits is by juicing. In addition to apple and carrot juicing, I would juice the cruciferous vegetables: cabbage, broccoli, Brussels sprouts, spinach, kale, cauliflower. These vegetables contain a chemical, Indole 3 Carbinol, that fights and helps heal breast cancer. Patients can also take Indole 3 Carbinol by capsule form (200 mg TID). I would take cabbage and broccoli on a regular basis, not only by juicing, but by meals. Look for recipes with cabbage and broccoli, Brussels sprouts, and spinach, in addition to apple and carrot juice. I would add Superfood Greens Plus, a blend of twenty-nine active enzymes that enhance and strengthen the immune system (echinacea, astragulus root, and probiotic cultures) with chlorophyll, which cleanses the colon gently; it also increases energy and mental acuity and emulsifies and metabolizes fats; add three scoops of the Greens Plus to eight ounces of juice, in addition to Indole 3 Carbinol. I would take vitamin D-3 hormone (5000 IU BID) to prevent or heal breast cancer.

Stress is caused by the adrenal hormone cortisol. DHEA can block cortisol. DHEA (25 mg) is recommended to control stress and depression for patients with breast cancer. When I was in medical practice, I referred my breast cancer patients to Dr. Simone and was very satisfied with the way he treated them. By the way, Dr. Simone was a strong proponent of exercise.

I recommend that my patients with breast cancer take a brisk walk of one to two miles daily and join a gym, and do yoga, aerobics, resistance exercises, and even Pilates. I strongly advise my patients not to take chemotherapy, radiation, or Tomoxophen.

CHAPTER 25

Emotional Freedom Techniques: Acupuncture without Needles

Emotional freedom techniques represent energy therapy; they are like acupuncture without needles. Using the eight acupuncture points, choose a specific problem, say anxiety. Give the anxiety a rating from 0 to 10. Perform a setup while tapping on the outside of the hand (karate chop); repeat this affirmation three times: "Even though I have this anxiety, I deeply and completely accept myself." Tap following points while repeating the reminder phrase:

- Eyebrow (EB)
- Side of eye (SE)
- Under the eye (UE)
- Under nose (UN)
- Chin (CH)
- Collarbone (CB)
- Underarm (UA)
- Head (H)

Rate the anxiety again from 0 to 10. Repeat the setup while tapping the outside of the hand; repeat the revised affirmation: "Even though I still have some of this anxiety, I deeply and completely accept myself."

Tap all the points again, repeating the revised reminder phrase.

Assess the rating again from 0 to 10. Repeat if necessary. Change to other problems.

EFT TREATMENT POINTS

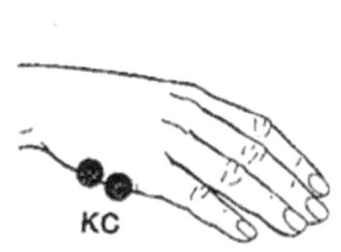

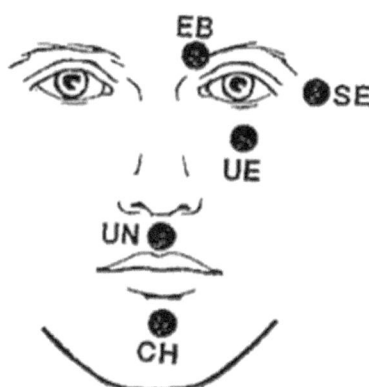

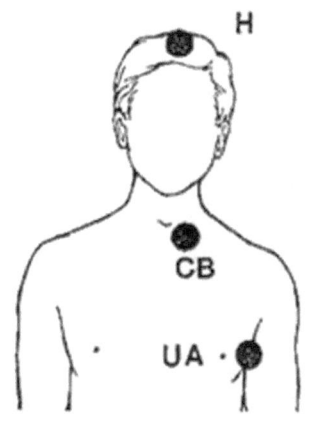

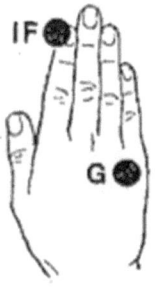

CHAPTER 26

2003 World Tour in 107 Days

In 2003, my wife, Virginia, and I traveled around the world on the *Queen Elizabeth II*. We departed from Fort Lauderdale and traveled for 107 days. We had daily lectures and daily dancing classes. We took computer classes and language classes in Italian, Spanish, French, and German.

We enjoyed going through the Panama Canal and visiting Panama City, where we had dinner and a folklore show. The costumes were magnificent, some costing as much as ten thousand dollars. The girls were beautiful. Next we went to Acapulco; the cliff divers were exciting. They climbed 135 feet and dove into 9 feet of water. After they dove, we took pictures with the divers. We went on to Los Angeles, where we joined my son and his wife and spent the day touring the city. We had a pleasant experience in Hawaii, where we visited Pearl Harbor, the Bishop Historical Museum, and Waikiki. In Waikiki, we took a tour of the oldest hotel near Diamond Head. Japanese couples often went to this hotel to get married. Except for the black pearls and the exhibition of the ship the *Bounty*, Tahiti was disappointing. But Morrea was one of the most beautiful islands that I have ever seen. The entire island was like a botanical garden.

The people of New Zealand were very friendly; the city was well organized and very clean. We viewed the entire city from a skytop building. Sailboats were everywhere; one in four people have sailboats. I enjoyed the New Zealand wines.

Australia was a highlight of the trip. I bought some wine in Tasmania and visited the army barracks and some old mansions. I never did see the Tasmanian devil.

Melbourne, a city of about three million people, was a place of trams. There were trams everywhere. My wife and I had lunch on a tram; we viewed the city by going to the Rialto Tower, fifty-four feet high. I had the opportunity to meet the relatives of the founder of Melbourne, Lord Melbourne. The city has a magnificent entertainment center with three theaters that seat a total of 6,000; the Greek population is very high, the highest next to Athens.

On the coast of Melbourne, there are thousands of kangaroos. Sydney was immaculate and friendly. Virginia and I visited the famed opera house, took a walk on the famous bridge, and later took a two-hour ferry ride on the harbor. We got a chance to see waterfront homes valued at $300,000 and more.

Next, we went to Brisbane, which was similar to the climate in Florida.

The most exciting part of my visit to Australia was the Great Barrier Reef at Cairns. The reef extends some 1,500 miles and consists of soft and hard coral. We boarded a submersible vessel and got a close-up view of the different shape coral and the multicolored fish. I even took a helicopter ride to view the reefs from 2,000 feet. In Brisbane, we saw the shearing of sheep.

Manila was a disaster, a poor country with many shacks with no running water or plumbing. There is a great disparity of poor from the 10 percent of families who are wealthy. There are a few families that have all the wealth in Manila.

Nagasaki, Japan, was a sad experience. We visited the Peace Park and the Atomic Museum. We got a firsthand look at the victims of the atomic bomb. There was an exhibition of the many people with radiation burns and those who developed leukemia and cancer. In Kyoto, we saw beautiful Shinto shrines and Buddhist temples. We ate lunch at a fine Japanese restaurant.

Hong Kong, the largest port in the world, was an enjoyable experience, particularly the tram ride to Victoria Peak, where we had the opportunity to view the skyscrapers of the city. We took a ride on a sampan in the Aberdeen section of Hong Kong. Lastly, we went to the Stanley Market for shopping.

We did not go to Kenya because of terrorism; instead we went to a French island, Reunion. Most of the coastal towns were named after saints.

The most beautiful beaches in the world were in the Seychelles. Because of the coral, the water has many shades of blue, and the sand is white. The hills are verdant, and in the water are granite peaks and round rocks. Tuna fishing is a source of income. They export tuna and red snapper. I saw a red snapper fourteen pounds in weight; we also went to Mauritius, an independent island, where 60 percent of the population is Indian. We visited an Indian market, a Hindu temple, and magnificent waterfalls.

I enjoyed my visit to Ho Chi Minh City. My wife and I went there on our own. We took a ninety-minute hydrofoil ride from the port. When we arrived in Saigon, we hired a taxi and were fortunate that the driver spoke English. He took us on a four-hour tour in a city of 2.4 million motorcycles. We visited Chinatown. The Rex Hotel was where the Americans were stationed during the war. We also went to the American War Museum. The exhibition at the museum was sad. The tragedy of war was also seen outside, as there were many war vehicles on display. We also visited the new Grand Hotel, the newest hotel. The hotel was noted for Chinese food.

We went to Singapore, which is another place that I would visit again. The second largest port after Hong Kong, Singapore has a population of 4.5 million; it is an immaculate city known for electronics. We visited the Rafters Hotel, the oldest hotel in the city. Virginia and I also went to the Oriental Hotel and met the manager, who was very cordial. The hotel is situated across from the marina and the financial center.

While we were in Singapore, our ship captain, Captain Warrick, left to take over the *Queen Mary II*. One evening, our group went to the newest hotel for Captain Warrick's going-away party. We had a wonderful dinner, entertainment, and dancing. I took pictures of Captain Warrick and his wife, Kim. I also met our new captain, Captain Wright.

Sri Lanka was a disaster, a very poor country. Most houses are shacks without water and plumbing. Most structures are bungalow style. The one thing that I did enjoy was the elephant orphanage, where we saw sixty elephants in one place, the largest collection in the world. We also went to a Buddhist temple that held one of the teeth of Buddha. There were also many gold Buddhas. We had lunch at the Regency Hotel in Candy.

We went on to Durban, South Africa, where there is 49 percent unemployment (mostly in the black population). Hundreds of thousands of blacks commute every day to the city and sell products on the street. The government has to clean the streets every night. It is a mess. The main city is very attractive, and the real estate is very reasonable.

Another place that I would return to is Cape Town, South Africa, a most beautiful city. The architecture is unique. Many of the buildings are white, and the botanical gardens are a sight to behold. The landmark is Table Mountain. We took a cable car to the top of the mountain and took pictures. The mountain is over 1,000 feet high. We also visited a museum and saw one of the most extensive collections of stuffed animals. There is much unemployment in Cape Town. Two million blacks live in shacks without running water or plumbing. I think Cape Town is a place to be reckoned with in the future. They are building a convention center.

The next day, we went to Shellenbosh and visited a winery, Morgandof. We saw how the wine was made. Then we had a wine tasting, followed by lunch. We drank an excellent Cabernet Sauvignon and Chenin Blanc. Shellenbosh is a university town of 100,000 inhabitants. We also took a tour of the old houses of the area. Shellenbosh is a place that I would like to return to and spend some more time. It was a very tranquil place.

Next we went to Saint Helena and visited the tomb of Napoleon, his home, Longwood, and his gardens. Napoleon lived there for six years. He died in 1821 from cancer of the stomach. While he was there, he took care of the gardens and played chess and billiards to pass time. He liked to read Homer's poems. He had an entourage of twenty-one people, including one of his generals.

Saint Helena was named after Emperor Constantine's mother. The island is poor, without an airport and with very few hotels. The average wage is forty to sixty dollars a week.

Next came Tenerife, Santa Cruz, a beautiful Spanish island (Canary Islands) with two golf courses. Mont Teide, a mountain of over 12,000 feet, is a landmark. The top of this volcanic mountain is covered with snow. The very irregularly shaped rock formations are a sight to behold, as well as the pine forest. The island imported ten million trees to Mount Teide. The climate is mild and the scenery is spectacular. The houses are multicolored. Our group had lunch at the El Monasterio. Spanish and English are spoken on the island. I tried to speak Spanish most of the time. Vino Blanco is the popular wine of the region. For lunch I was hoping for seafood paella, but instead I got roasted chicken.

Because of the bad weather, we did not go to the Portuguese island, Madeira; instead, we went to Vigo, Spain. It was another opportunity for me to speak Spanish. Vigo is a town in the north of Spain.

We visited Santiago de Compostela; next to Rome and Jerusalem, it is the holiest Catholic site in the world. The tomb of St. James the Apostle is at the cathedral of Santiago de Compostela. It is the most famous place for pilgrimages since the Middle Ages, dating from AD 900. I attended mass and had the privilege of taking a picture with the cardinal.

CHAPTER 27

Lifestyle Degenerative Diseases Can Be Prevented

I am excited. I am here to educate and make a difference, put myself on the line. We now can prevent some sixty lifestyle degenerative diseases and conditions, such as heart disease, stroke, cancer, diabetes, arthritis, autoimmune diseases, lupus, chronic fatigue syndrome, fibromyalgia, MS, ALS, migraine, carpal tunnel, osteoporosis, spina bifida, Alzheimer's, and Parkinson's. Although we can't stop aging, we can slow it down.

These diseases can be prevented because we know the cause. We want to get to the cause, not suppress the symptoms. Conventional medicine treats healing like it was a leaking faucet: it has been cleaning up the wet floor instead of shutting off the faucet. The body heals itself, and as Hippocrates said, "First, do no harm."

The cause is the free radicals. What are the free radicals? The free radicals are unstable molecules of oxygen, missing one electron. They become bandits, stealing electrons from healthy cells and converting them into free radicals, causing a chain reaction, even putting holes in the cell membranes, gaining entrance into the DNA, causing mutations, cancer, lipid peroxidation, and oxidative damage. The only way we can neutralize and devitalize these free radicals is by taking antioxidants such as angiotensin-converting enzyme (ACE), selenium, chelated minerals, and proflavanol (grape seed extract, bioflavonoids).

One can observe the free radicals in our environment; when you cut an apple and expose it to air, it becomes discolored; similarly, fats turn rancid in air, iron gates rust, windshield wipers wrinkle and don't work properly. These degenerative, lifestyle diseases are caused by the same process.

What is the source of these free radicals? Where do they come from? They come from air, food, water, and stress. In the air, we have carbon dioxide, ozone, industrial pollutants, viruses, bacteria, allergens, and smoke (use an air ionizer that supplies negative ions or an electronic air cleaner for indoor air pollution; I recommend Enviracaire from Honeywell, which is recommended by the American Lung Association). Much of our food is contaminated by insecticides, pesticides, hormones, and antibiotics—more antibiotics than the medical profession uses (use organically grown food free from pesticides, hormones, and antibiotics). Much of our water is unclean, polluted by chlorine, bacteria such as e. coli, and toxic metals (use reverse osmosis filter or bottled water for clean water). Stress aggravates the effects of free radicals on the body. Learn to handle stress and employ the relaxation response, meditation, self-hypnosis, breathing and relaxation exercises, mindfulness, yoga, or prayer.

The body produces free radicals and also produces antioxidants. Each cell has antioxidants, enzymes like superoxide desmutase, catalase, glutathione peroxidase, and glutathione reductase (enzymes are catalysts and speed up a chemical reaction).

We now know the cause, the source, and the solution of lifestyle degenerative diseases. The cause is free radicals; the source is pollution; and the solution is antioxidants. Health is a state of physical, mental (thoughts), emotional (feelings), and spiritual (energy, consciousness, creative imagination) well-being.

Every belief system needs references or legs. I like to use the metaphor of a table with four legs; the table top, representing health, is supported by four legs:

Leg 1. A healthy diet: low fat, complex carbs, and high fiber
Leg 2. Nutritional supplements, herbs, and chelated minerals
Leg 3. Physical exercise
Leg 4. Mental exercise

Leg 1: A healthy diet requires grains, fruits, vegetables, legumes, garlic, onions, nuts, cold water fish, and eight to ten glasses of clean water daily. Grains: oatmeal with berries or bananas. Fresh fruit: water-containing fruits such as watermelon, cantaloupe, oranges, apples, pears, and plums are rich in antioxidants. Fresh organic veggies (antioxidants): broccoli, cabbage, spinach, carrots (each carrot contains 6 mg of beta-carotene), Brussels sprouts, eggplants. Legumes: beans, lentils, white and red kidney beans, black beans, rice, and pasta (lima beans are a good protein source, low in fat and high in fiber). Cold-water fish (high in omega 3 and 6): salmon, sardines, halibut, mackerel, and herring. Use canola oil or extra virgin olive oil. Flax seed oil can be used on salads.

We can get antioxidants in our diets if we get at least five servings of fruits and vegetables daily. How many of us actually get five servings of each every day? Not many; even if we did, there is no way you would get enough of the antioxidants needed just through diet.

Supplementation is the answer, but researchers at the National Cancer Institute found that the regular multiple supplements do not contain enough antioxidants to confer a benefit.

Leg 2: Supplements and herbs. Because of degraded food, insecticides, pesticides, hormones, and antibiotics, we need supplements. The soil in Florida, for example, lacks zinc and selenium.

Good nutrition requires proper cell nourishment, the right nutrients, the right concentration, the right balance, all readily available to the cell. Nutrition is also based on synergy: all B vitamins work together, vitamin E works with selenium, zinc works with copper, B6 and C work together.

Nutrition depends on lifestyle: avoid concentrated sugar, caffeine, nicotine, alcohol, and milk. Finally, renewal is important: all cells renew themselves. We form a new stomach lining in five days, a new liver in six weeks, new skin in 28 days, and new red blood cells in 120 days. By the end of one year, we have a new body.

Dr. Myron Wentz, famed virologist and immunologist, developed the diagnostic tests for the Epstein-Barr virus and the herpes virus. In cell cultures that Dr. Wentz has grown over the last twenty years, he found that human cells could survive indefinitely if carefully given the right nutrients and an environment protected from toxins. After Dr. Wentz became ill, he went to pharmacies looking for vitamins. When he scientifically tested the products, he was astonished to find that many of the products were mislabeled. Some vitamins labeled 500 mg of vitamin C had only 50 mg. There was no control. So he decided to manufacture his own vitamins based on cellular technology and guaranteed the amount of the ingredients. His company is called USANA, which means "true health." Dr. Wentz is a dedicated scientist utilizing the latest research.

Dr. Michael Colgan, world-renowned sports nutritionist and author of the best-selling book *Optimum Sports Nutrition*, states, "In my more than twenty years in nutrition research, I've not seen a wellness program as impressive as that developed by Myron Wentz."

Dr. Randy Thompson, director of the Wellness Center at Washington State University, is a USANA advisory board member; he states, "USANA provides the most comprehensive program I have ever seen." USANA's comprehensive program consists of mega-antioxidants; chelated minerals; grape seed extract (proflavanol); poly C; calcium, magnesium, vitamin D, and boron; and Fibergy. The grape seed extract, proflavanol, is the world's most potent antioxidant: fifty times as potent as vitamin E and twenty times as potent as vitamin C. It remains in the body for twenty-four hours and enhances the action of vitamins E and C.

Poly C is a special form of vitamin C with calcium, magnesium, potassium, and zinc ascorbate. The product is easy on the GI tract and maintains a higher blood level of vitamin C.

The Life Extension Foundation in Hollywood, Florida, is another fine organization. It is the ultimate source for new health and medical findings from around the world. They also have an excellent vitamin formula called Life Extension Mix.

One can become a member of USANA or Life Extension and purchase the vitamins wholesale.

In addition to the antioxidants and chelated minerals, every cell needs flaxseed oil: organic cold pressed (1000 mg cap daily) or two tablespoonfuls of oil daily. Cells also need coenzyme Q10: this is a vitaminlike cofactor, a powerful antioxidant that strengthens the heart muscle, prevents heart failure, and boosts energy levels. It also lowers blood pressure.

I would be remiss not to mention garlic, which lowers BP and cholesterol, thins the blood, and helps regulate the sugar. It has antibacterial, antifungal, and anticancer effects (4000 mg Enzymatic daily).

What studies show the value of the antioxidants? The American Heart Association gave 90,000 women vitamin E for two years, and their risk of cardiovascular disease was cut 50 percent. A Harvard study gave men sixty-five years of age and under vitamin E for two years, and heart disease was cut 50 percent. There was a study done in China with over 3,500 people taking antioxidants and minerals for a ten-year period, with an amazing 38 percent reduction in cardiovascular disease. There is an inverse relationship between vitamin E and heart disease. The higher the blood level of vitamin E, the less the heart disease. For example, in Finland, where they consume a lot of fat in their diet, there is a high incidence of heart disease, and the level of vitamin E in the blood is low.

The levels of minerals and vitamins found in our foods have drastically declined. For example, in 1948 spinach had 158 mg of iron per 100 gm. In 1997, spinach has an average iron content of 2.2 mg per 100 gm. That means you would have to eat seventy-five bowls of spinach today to get the same amount of iron that you got in the days of Popeye.

According to the *RDA Handbook*, we are eating empty foods: 50 to 70 percent of vitamin B6 is lost in meat processing; 50 to 90 percent is lost in milling cereals; 50 percent of folic acid may be lost during processing and storage; 80 percent of magnesium is lost by removal of the germ and outer layers of cereal grains.

Is your vitamin supplement adequate? According to Dr. Michael Colgan in his book *The New Nutrition*, the major brands lack adequate levels of vitamins. Capitalizing on the mass of new evidence, ads for many foods say, "Contains the complete antioxidant group." That may be true, but in what amounts?

When you read the small print on the label, it may say it has 60 mg of vitamin C, yet studies show that we need 2000 to 3000 mg; for vitamin E, the label may say 30 IU, yet studies show that disease-prevention effects of vitamin E require 400 to 800 IU.

In the early 1900s, the leading causes of premature death were diphtheria, influenza, tuberculosis, and pneumonia. These are all infectious diseases.

In 1997, the leading causes of premature death were heart disease, cancer, stroke, and diabetes. All are man-made, lifestyle-based, degenerative diseases. What happened from 1900 to 1997? Planet earth has become polluted. Air, food, and water are polluted, and stress has increased as well. The environment is more toxic and unsafe; nutrients in our food supply are depleted; commercial fertilizers are overused; foods are overprocessed and preserved; the water supply is contaminated and unclean; and our fast-paced, stressful lifestyle is slowly killing us.

Now, let us go to the third leg of health: physical exercise. Dr. Colgan states, "The right exercise is a major strategy for preventing and treating all disease." There is evidence that moderate exercise strengthens your immunity. It increases lymphocytes, neutrophiles (white blood cells), and interleukin-2. Exercise can prevent cancer, lower cholesterol, protect blood pressure, strengthen the heart and lungs, increase vital capacity, and lower blood sugar (which helps with diabetes, prevents osteoporosis, and is of tremendous value in decreasing depression).

Brisk walking is the ideal exercise. If one has arthritis, then swimming or walking in the water are recommended. For knee problems, the stationary bicycle is preferred. Other forms of exercise include the treadmill, trampoline, and dancing.

Exercise in the morning and pick an area relatively free from pollution. One should aim to do two miles in thirty minutes, three miles in forty-five minutes. To figure the ideal heart rate, Dr. Michael Murray suggests that you subtract your age from 185. For example, I am 75 years of age; my target rate would be 110 beats per minute; subtract 20 from this figure to get the lowest range. For me, it would be 90. While exercising, use the carotid artery in the neck in order to determine the heart rate. Place your index and middle finger at the angle of the jaw and move the fingers to the neck region, count for six seconds and add a zero. For example, if your beats were 11 in six seconds, add a zero and your rate per minute would be 110.

Attempt to work up a sweat, and after exercising use some resistive exercises, using mild weights. Remember, fats burn in muscle; preserve your muscles. For weight reduction, your goal should be to lose one pound a week in order to keep the weight off.

And avoid the yo-yo phenomenon (losing and gaining back weight). The latest research shows that we should lose weight slowly. Exercise one body part per week, except for the abdominals. Chest and back one day, then legs (quads and hamstrings), shoulder, and arms (biceps and triceps); work on your abdominals four times a week.

Remember, being overweight is an illness, and cancer, heart disease, and diabetes love body fat. Keep the fat calories down to 20 percent; measure body fat once a month. Fat calories are high: 1 gram of fat is equal to 9 calories, while carbs and protein are 4 calories per gram.

Now, let us proceed to the fourth leg: mental exercise (relaxation exercises).

Recent studies attribute 85 percent of all disease to stress-related factors. In America, fourteen million people suffer from anxiety and 30 percent suffer from chronic to severe insomnia. The major factors are unhealthy lifestyle and attitude: helplessness and hopelessness; low self-esteem; not having a loving, worthwhile, and capable attitude; isolation (Dean Ornish, in his book *Reversing Heart Disease*, attributes isolation as a big causative factor); and deprivation.

When the body is under stress, the nervous system responds by increasing sympathetic activity. The blood pressure goes up, pulse rises, blood sugar goes up, muscles tighten, the bronchial tubes open, allowing more oxygen, preparing the organism for flight or fight. This damages the body and can lead to heart disease and diabetes. Prolonged stress results in release of cortisol and ultimately glucose depletion, burn out, and adrenal insufficiency. This is the so-called stress response.

The opposite is the relaxation response popularized by Dr. Herbert Benson of Harvard. The parasympathetic autonomic nervous system is responsible for relaxation. The relaxation technique uses a mantra or sound. The stress response was popularized by Dr. Hans Selye of Canada.

There are many techniques for relaxation. The bottom line is focal concentration. To mention a few, yoga, creative visualization, progressive muscular relaxation, mindfulness prayer (meditation), and breathing exercises.

I would like to concentrate on breathing exercises for relaxation. Diaphragmatic breathing is a must for relaxation. The diaphragm is a dome-shaped muscle that lies between the chest cavity and the abdominal cavity. When you breathe in, the diaphragm rises to allow more oxygen in, and when you exhale, the diaphragm drops, allowing the carbon dioxide and wastes to escape. Have you ever noticed how a baby breathes? With each breath, the baby's abdomen rises and falls. Most adults use chest breathing, which does not use the diaphragm; the result is shallow breathing, which produces tension and fatigue.

When you learn to breathe with the diaphragm, you will notice more energy and less stress. It takes practice. How do you learn to breathe with the diaphragm?

Find a comfortable, quiet place to sit. Place your feet slightly apart. Place one hand on your abdomen near your navel. Place the other hand on your chest. You will be inhaling through your nose and exhaling through your mouth. Concentrate on your breathing. Note which hand is rising and falling with each breath.

I would like to present a breathing exercise that only takes a few minutes; you could do it several times a day for any purpose you so desire, any stressful situation.

Gently exhale most of the air in your lungs. Let go completely. Now, deeply inhale through your nose; with mouth and eyes closed, count to 4 and as you inhale, allow your abdomen to rise an inch. Make sure that you are not moving your chest or shoulders. As you breathe in the warm air, the oxygen will be flowing to all the cells in your body. Hold your breath for the count of 7; this allows more oxygen to get into the tissues. Then slowly exhale for the count of 8. Your abdomen should move inward. The exhalation should be two times the inhalation. Prolonged exhalation gets rid of the waste and cellular debris; the lymph system is responsible for the waste products; unlike the heart, the lymph system does not have a pump and requires breathing for movement.

This exercise does three things: 1. relaxation, 2. increase oxygenation, and 3. remove waste and carbon dioxide. Throughout the entire exercise, place your thumb and index and middle fingers together, creating a circle (circuit). One other point: the ultimate in concentration is to focus on one idea or task. With this exercise, you are focusing on breathing only. How many times should you do this exercise and when is the best time? In the beginning, do the exercise four times (four cycles) and then increase it to eight times. The best time is in the morning, and the second best time is at bedtime. To prolong exhalation, puckering your lips is helpful.

Every night when I go to bed, I ask myself, what did I learn? When you go to bed tonight, I want you to ask yourself the same question. We learned that free radicals are the cause of lifestyle degenerative diseases, the source is pollution, and the solution is the antioxidants in food and supplements. We learned that we are what we breathe: clean air (use an indoor electronic filter); we are what we eat: organic foods; we are what we drink: clean water (use a reverse osmosis filter); and we are what we think: if I think I can, my unconscious will accept it and carry it out. If I think I can't, my unconscious will carry it out.

We learned that health is a state of physical, mental, emotional, and spiritual well-being, and it depends on the four legs of health: a healthy diet, nutritional supplements, physical exercises, and mental exercises. We learned that we can prevent these lifestyle degenerative diseases—heart disease, stroke, cancer, diabetes, arthritis—because the cause is the same: the free radicals. Finally, participate in your healthcare with your conventional doctor for diagnosis (technology), surgery, and acute emergencies, which is 20 percent of the time. The other 80 percent of the time, after a diagnosis is made, use natural medicine that helps the body heal, does no harm, and treats the cause. My mission in life is to integrate alternative medicine with conventional medicine. Your mission should be the same.

CHAPTER 28
Heart Disease

One million people die annually from heart disease. The good news is heart disease can be prevented and can be reversed, even if you have coronary disease. History is important, particularly if your mother or father died of heart disease before age fifty. A physical exam can help detect cardiac problems such as heart failure, angina, hypertension, arrhythmia, heart block, valvular heart disease, and heart muscle abnormalities. Annual blood tests are important to assess chemzyme plus, CBC, urine, lipid profile, thyroid profile including TSH, homocysteine, coenzyme Q10, and fibrinogen blood levels.

Heart disease is a lifestyle degenerative disease caused by free radicals and can be prevented with antioxidants, which neutralize the free radicals. According to Dr. Stephen T. Sinatra, eminent cardiologist, there is no reason to have heart disease today.

Presently, the fat-cholesterol theory for atherosclerosis is the most popular. It states that the free radicals oxidize the low-density lipoprotein cholesterol in the endothelium, the lining of the coronary vessels; foam cells (fat cells) are formed and the macrophages (large white blood cells) engulf the foam cells and become overstuffed, allowing fat cells along with sticky platelets to adhere to the lining, causing plaque formation and atherosclerosis. So the very oxygen that is necessary for life is also a villain, causing oxidative damage to the coronaries. For decades, we have been taught that cholesterol is the culprit.

In 1948, the Framingham Heart Study was done to determine the cause of atherosclerotic heart disease. Researchers in Framingham, Massachusetts, a suburb of Boston, enrolled 5,209 local residents, ranging in age from thirty to sixty-two. They were examined every two years. In 1970, 5,135 adult offspring of the original participants joined the study. As a result of this study, the cardiovascular risk factors were born, a term coined by Dr. William Kannel, the first director of the Framingham Study. Dr. Kannel said the major risk factors that can be changed are elevated serum cholesterol, cigarette smoking, and hypertension. Other risk factors include obesity, diabetes, glucose intolerance, sedentary lifestyle, stress (type A personality), and elevated fibrinogen blood levels. Recently, elevated homocysteine has been added to the list as an independent risk factor. The protective factors are HDL and exercise.

The Framingham Study emphasized that for every 1 percent drop in cholesterol, there is a 2 percent decrease in cardiovascular disease (that is a decrease in the LDL cholesterol, bad cholesterol). For every 1 percent rise in HDL (good cholesterol), there is a 3 percent decrease in cardiovascular disease. The multiple risk factor intervention trial showed that drugs offer no benefit against heart disease in borderline to moderate hypertension.

In my way of thinking, stress is a major risk factor that most physicians neglect. *Is It Worth Dying For?* by Dr. Robert S. Eliot explains how to make stress work for you, not against you. Cardiologist Dr. Dean Ornish (author of *Reversing Heart Disease*) also believes that stress is a major risk factor.

In Dr. Ornish's famous lifestyle heart trial, he divided his patients into a control and experimental group. The experimental group was asked to perform stress-reduction techniques such as breathing exercises, stretching exercises, meditation, imagery, and other relaxation regimens for one hour a day and to exercise at least three times weekly. In addition they were placed on a diet of grains, fruits and veggies, legumes, and soy products. No animal products were allowed except egg whites, one cup of nonfat milk, or yogurt. The diet consisted of 10 percent fat, 20 percent protein, and 70 percent complex carbohydrates.

At the end of a year, the experimental group showed overall regression of atherosclerosis, while the control group, following the American Heart Association's diet, actually showed progression of their disease. Dr. Sinatra considers 10 percent saturated fat too low. He favors a 20 to 25 percent fat regimen. Dr. Murray feels that a strict vegetarian diet, advocated by Dr. Ornish, may not be as important as diet high in fiber and complex carbohydrates and low in fat and cholesterol. However, a vegetarian diet has been shown to be quite effective in lowering cholesterol and reducing the risk of atherosclerosis.

Anger and hostility can activate the sympathetic nervous system with a release of adrenalin, resulting in a rise in blood pressure and pulse, clotting of blood, elevation of blood sugar, and opening of the bronchial tubes, allowing more oxygen to enter the cardiovascular system, preparing the individual for flight or fight. This is the so-called stress response developed by Hans Selye.

Free radicals and environmental pollution can trigger heart disease, while antioxidants such as coenzyme Q10, with the help of L-Carnitine diet, exercise, and a healthy lifestyle, can prevent heart disease. Antioxidants are the key to the prevention of heart disease.

CHAPTER 29

The Mind

The mind is a form of energy.
—Candice Pert.

My Mind
My mind is a builder;
My mind and brain are one–the mind-brain.
My mind builds reality.
My mind builds the future.
My mind is in my body.
My mind is in my brain.

The brain is made of three parts:

1. The brain stem
2. The cerebellum
3. The cerebrum

The cerebral cortex is the storehouse of my thoughts. I can hold a human brain in my hand; it weighs three pounds. I can't hold my mind in my hand, because it is energy. My brain is involved in everything I do. My mind also works incessantly. I am a silent witness to my thoughts. I am a silent witness to moments of emptiness. Nothingness is everythingness. I am a silent witness to the sacred space between my thoughts, where my creativity is, where God is, where my cosmic consciousness resides. While I am taking a deep breath through my nose, there are no thoughts. My being is still and peaceful. My being does nothing. I am whole, and my mind, body, and spirit emerge.

ROAD TO HEALING AND CURING BREAST CANCER

ANTHONY ALOSI, M.D

TABLE OF CONTENTS

INTRODUCTION

Ninety percent of all cancers are related to nutritional factors. The nutritional factors for breast cancer are high animal fat, low fiber, smoking, alcohol, high cholesterol and environmental pollution. According to the World Health Organization, health is a state of physical, mental, emotional and spiritual well being. When we travel on the road we come to a fork in the road, on the right breast cancer benefits from the hormone vitamin D3. Vitamin D3 prevents fifty to sixty percent of breast cancers; also Indole 3 Carbinol prevents breast cancer.

Broccoli, cabbage, Brussels sprouts, kale and cauliflower prevent breast cancer, because of the Indole-3 Carbinol in these foods. Curcumin and Selenium are also anti-cancer minerals. Every morning for fifteen years, I took greens plus powder plus 18x Aloe Vera. Recently blueberry was added. I take three scoops in eight ounces of apple juice, plus one ounce of 18x Aloe Vera. For stress I would take complete Dhea (one capsule – Life Extension Brand. On the left side of the road, I would eliminate Tomoxaphen, and radiation (radiation causes cancer).

I would eliminate chemotherapy which is toxic in my opinion. The ideal surgery is lumpectomy with axilary and suplavicular lymph gland removal. The lymph glands are full of white blood cells. I would be remiss not to mention my relationship with Dr Charles B Simeone, author of "Cancer Nutrition." When I was in practice I referred my breast cancer patients to Dr Simeone who did a wonderful job.

What is cancer? Cancer cells divide in an uncontrolled disorganized fashion. Oncogenes cause the initiation, promotion and spread of cancer. There is disorganization; undifferentiating and mutation in the DNA, there are also Repressor P53 genes that prevent cancer. Every cancer patient benefits from exercise, walking, yoga, Pilates, mindfulness meditation and abdominal exercises.

The seven level program involves doing and being. The program is designed to answer the relative and ultimate purposes of medicine. The relative purpose is to relieve symptoms and cure the cancer. With respect to cancer the purpose of medicine is to eradicate the tumor, normalize the blood studies, relieve pain, clear the CT scans and prolong life. The ultimate purpose of medicine is to assist all beings to experience love, joy and peace and to know who we really are. The program begins with a discussion of the basics: State-of-the-art medical care.

Level one: Education and information about cancer particularly breast and current treatment options. This empowers patients to actively participate in their care.

Level two: Psychosocial support explores the importance of reaching out to others in the journey through cancer breast cancer groups to heal.

In level three: the body as garden, patients and family members are invited to see the human body as a growing and evolving whole. A living garden rather than a machine. This level explores diet, good nutrition, supplements, herbs, exercise, massage, relaxation and stress management and other complementary and alternative approaches to healing.

Level four: Emotional healing enters the inner realm of the heart. Emotional healing includes the healing power of self-love and forgiveness. Express your feelings on a daily basis by means of a journal.

Level five: The nature of mind looks carefully at how our entire experience of life (including life with cancer) is determined by our thoughts, our beliefs and the meaning we give to events.

Level six: Life assessment explores the hopes, goals and purposes of our lives. What we are. Living Fortis, the purpose of life is to be happy and have peace of mind. What do we want to share with others while we are alive regardless of how long we live?

Level seven: The nature of spirit embraces the spiritual aspects of the healing process, as well as the dimension of our being that exists beyond illness, beyond even birth and death.

THE BASICS: STATE-OF-THE-ART MEDICAL CARE

For the present the conventional doctor employs surgery, radiation and chemotherapy. Surgery has changed from the early days from radical mastectomy, partial mastectomy until the present lumpectomy. Today the tumor is removed with the surrounding tissue even the lymph nodes in the axilla (under the arms) are carefully dissected, studied and removed. There has been improvement in radiation therapy. Chemotherapy has become more sophisticated with fewer side effects including the use of growth factors and stem cell transplantation.

Furthermore, the human genome project, which involves the mapping of three billion units of encoded genetic information contained in every human cell, is expected to be completed in the first half of the new century. New developments in gene therapy, immunotherapy and other emerging fields may soon race far ahead of current treatments. Doctors have been successfully using tumor-suppressor genes which can function effectively in forestalling cancer growth. The suppressor gene is called P-53; the body also has Oncogenes which promote the growth of cancer cells. Chemical agents and fat can activate the Oncogenes and initiate cancer growth. Cancer is a process that can take ten to forty years to develop. Once the process is initiated, the can progress and eventually spread, metastasize. Dr. Stanislaw Burzynski M.D., PhD has developed peptides which he called anti-neoplastons which have the ability to turn off the Oncogenes and stimulate the activity of the suppressor genes P53. He has successfully cured brain cancer and claims that it works in fifty percent of other cancers including breast cancer. New research on DNA damage and repair, angiogenesis, the ability of tumors to generate blood vessels which are necessary to provide themselves with vital nutrients – shark cartilage works by angiogenesis is on-going.

Recognize that fear, anxiety and depression are natural. A message in the book that I strongly agree with is that the mental, emotional and spiritual aspects of cancer are as important—if not more so—than the physical concerns.

Ask yourself this question? Do I have trust and confidence in my doctor? 1-your doctor should do no harm 2-your doctor should love you as much as himself, and treat you as he would a member of his own family. Recognize that your body needs love and attention, but so do your mind, heart and spirit.

The World Health Organization defines health as a state of physical, mental, emotional and spiritual well being. Unfortunately, the conventional doctor is trained to put all the attention on the body, but we have a mind and body and they influence each other.

Cancer questions and answers:

WHAT IS CANCER?

Cancer is uncontrolled abnormal growth of cancer cells. What causes cancer? In the DNA there are cancer-causing genes (Oncogenes) and there are genes that suppress cancer and protect us from getting cancer. These genes are called tumor suppressor genes. Cancer is initiated by chemicals, radiation and viruses. The pollutants and free radicals promote cancer. The pollutants are air, insecticides, pesticides, antibiotics, hormones in food, the heavy metals in the water, (lead, mercury cadmium and negative chemicals), adrenalin and cortisol caused by stress. Most experts agree that the pollution causes free radicals. While oxygen is necessary, it has a downside. Unstable oxygen missing one electron (negative charge) is the culprit. Free radicals are very important and cause oxidative damage and are responsible for degenerative diseases such as heart disease, stroke, cancer diabetes, arthritis, chronic fatigue, auto-immune disease Parkinsonism and Alzheimer's.

Free radicals are oxygen molecules missing one electrical charge (electron) as a result they become bandits, scavengers and steal electrons from other cell. They put holes in the cell membranes and get into the DNA and cause damage ultimately leading to cancer. It is a chain reaction each cell becomes a free radical until the cells are neutralized by antioxidants.

Antioxidants such as beta-carotene-vitamin E, vitamin C, selenium, grape seed extract and COQ10 neutralize the free radicals. Antioxidants and a strong immune system prevent relapse in cancer of the breast.

All cancers involve abnormal cells that divide in an uncontrolled disordered manner. These cancer cells have the capacity to spread from point of origin to other sites, this process is called metastasis.

A good metaphor is a wild forest fire that is out of control and spreads. Oncogenes are cancer producing genes in the DNA and are activated by chemicals, radiation and viruses. These carcinogenic agents initiate the cancer process. Alcohol, hormones (estrogen in breast cancer) polyunsaturated fats promote cancer. According to Dr, Charles Simione in his book "Cancer and Nutrition" only 2 alcoholic drinks a week increases cancer risk four fold. Also in the DNA are suppressor genes which block the cancer producing genes. Cancer is a process and takes years to progress and spread. There has been a marked increase in the estrogen sensitive breast cancers, while the estrogen insensitive cancers have not increased. In 1900, breast cancer in women was 20 to l. In 1976 breast cancer was 14 to 1 and in 2002 breast cancer increased to 1 in 8.

HOW DOES BREAST CANCER HARM THE BODY?

Cancer cells reproduce and form large tumors which may displace normal tissue in the case of the liver it can cause liver failure and in the lung it can cause obstruction of the airway. Cancer cells can obstruct the lymph channels and cause considerable swelling, damage nerves and muscles. It can also harm the body by raising calcium.

Metastatic cancer is difficult to control because it spreads from its primary site and may not be detectable, but often it maintains its original identity. Cancer spreads though the blood stream and lymphatic system. Breast cancer can spread to the lungs and is not lung cancer, but lung metastasis of breast cancer. It can spread to bones, particularly the pelvis, lumbar, spine, hips and ribs. It shows up as increased bone density called Osteoblastic Mets.

What are the main groups of cancers?

Carcinoma, sarcoma and leukemia/lymphomas are the most common. Carcinomas involve the glands such as the breast and prostate. When the breast gland becomes involved it is called Adenocarcinoma of the breast and are solid.

Tumor stage is most important in determining treatment:

Stage 1 – Tumors localized to the ducts: they do not spread and are 100% curable

Stage 2 – Tumors in general have spread only to the immediately surrounding tissues

Stage 3 – Tumors in general have spread a bit further than stage 2 tumors, and often involve nearby lymph nodes, usually the axillary (under the armpits)

Stage 4 – Tumors are those that have spread widely, including to other organs. The most common staging system is called TNM staging system. T refers to the size of the Tumor, N refers to whether or not lymph nodes are involved; and M refers to whether or not the cancer has metastasized to other organs or tissues

WHAT ARE TUMOR MARKERS?

Tumor markers are specialized proteins in the blood stream; the tumor marker for breast cancer is CA 15-3. The current treatment for breast cancer is surgery-lumpectomy and selective removal of the lymph nodes-to prevent Lymphedema (swelling of arm) today, radiation is applied using sophisticated techniques guided by advanced computer programs, which focus only on the tumor cells. Another is seed implants into the tumor. A specialized new form of radiation therapy is called Gamma-Knife Radiosurgery. A third type is called chemotherapy usually by intravenous route or oral medication.

HOW COMMON IS BREAST CANCER?

In 1999, four major types of cancer accounted for 50% of cancers. Cancer is second only to heart disease and prostate cancer is now number 1. Prostate cancer has reached epidemic proportions. Prostate 179,000 cases, Breast-176,000 cases – in 2002 breast cancer is 1 in 8 (in 1900 it was 1 in 21) lung – 172,000 cases. Colorectal cancer – 130,000 cases. A total of 657,000 out of 1.2 million overall.

What are the important issues in breast cancer?

Breast cancer is one of the most readily treatable cancers in humans. A number of risk factors have been recognized. Age is important as incidence increases over 50. A family history of breast cancer is associated with a higher predisposition to developing the disease. Early menstruation is a risk factor (age 12). Menses at age 16 is less of a risk. Increased exposure to estrogens over the years increases the chance of developing breast cancer. High fat in the diet and abdominal obesity increases estrogen. Estrogen causes cancer (Dr. Michael Colgan, "Hormonal Health")

The huge nurses study trial by researchers at Harvard Medical School followed 70,000 postmenopausal nurses for 10 years. Results have just been confirmed again what we knew 30 years ago. After five years of therapy with estrogen alone or estrogen plus progestin, risk of breast cancer increased 32%. A good chunk of the increase in breast cancer in postmenopausal women in America has estrogen therapy as its root cause.

Risk of breast cancer increases in women who have a pregnancy after thirty. Risk of breast cancer increases with alcohol consumption (3 studies). Two drinks a week increases risk four fold. It is wise not to drink alcohol. Exercise is helpful in reducing risk of breast cancer in women and this is related to a decrease in estrogens.

Walking is the best exercise. Start thirty minutes and gradually increase to an hour. Brisk walking is more beneficial. Other exercises are swimming, bicycle riding and dancing. Exercise about four to six a week. Evidence suggest low fat (saturated and solid fats should be eliminated) plant based diets of fruit and veggies, legumes and grains offer protection. According to Professor Lewis Thomas, President of

Sloan Kettering Cancer Hospital, the human body is incredibly tough given the right nutrition, exercise and lifestyle; it will resist cancer for a lifetime.

Eminent Biostaticlan Dr. Ulrich Abel cites poll after poll of cancer physicians showing that many would refuse chemotherapy if they developed cancer themselves. Lumpectomy is still surgical treatment of choice along with selective lymph node removal and sophisticated radiation treatments. According to Dr. Michael Colgan, the new nutrition, we need more than the standard chemotherapy, surgery and radiation. Nutrition, exercise and lifestyle changes are a must, not only tumor reduction, but treatment of the whole person from the inside. Dr. LaBriola, a cancer specialist, believes that in addition to conventional treatments the patient should employ many of the natural strategies that are available. In other words there should be a marriage between conventional and complementary medicine.

Neal Barnard M.D. makes a strong case for a low fat, vegetarian diet with exercise for breast cancer patients in his book "Eat Right Live Longer". As we have seen, foods exert a powerful influence over hormones, and hormones play a decisive role in breast cancer. Asian countries such as Japan, which have traditionally followed diets based on rice, vegetables, soy with little meat or dairy products, have had very low breast cancer rates. Foods not only help prevent cancer, they can also improve survival for those who have breast cancer. The more the diet is plant-based and the lower the fat content, the better the odds. In general, vegetable-rich plant-based diets improve survival rate while alcohol reduces the survival odds, reducing body weight also helps. Several studies have shown that slimmer women live longer with cancer than women with more body fat.

Currently, the method of detection of breast cancer is still self exam and mammography over age 50 (GE-Sonogram-Improvement) again breast cancer is one of the most treatable, if not always curable diseases.

LEVEL TWO-PSYCHOSOCIAL SUPPORT

Connection with other people lies at the heart of healing. Strong scientific evidence now shows that love and support from others translates into better health, not just emotional but physical as well. Personally, I have found that when I have a problem and there is no solution, love and support helps. Support groups relieve the overwhelming sense of isolation experienced by the cancer patients.

In a landmark study published in the medical journal The Lancet, Dr. David Spiegel demonstrated that women with breast cancer who received social and emotional support, in addition to receiving the standard medical care had less anxiety, depression and pain than women who received no such support. Even more astonishingly, the women who received the extra support lived on the average more than twice as long. The results were published by Dr. Spiegel in 1989 in his study, "Eighty-Six Women with Metastatic Breast Cancer". The subjects were randomly assigned to two groups, who met once a week for 90 minutes for one year.

Dr. Spiegel in his book "Living Beyond Limits" mentions how surprised he was that the support group lived twice as long. I had the pleasure several years ago of meeting Dr. Spiegel in Philadelphia. At that time, he reported that the support group lived 36.6 months compared with 18.9 months for the women who did not participate. He also taught the group self-hypnosis. The self-hypnosis was very effective in relieving anxiety and pain.

TYPES OF SUPPORT GROUPS

Open ended groups are probably the most common setting for psychosocial support in cancer. Groups may include family members, friends, and caregivers. Typically groups meet on a regular basis with social workers, clinicians or even former patients acting as facilitators. Although patients may initially feel apprehensive about joining a support group, the vast majority find the experience beneficial in terms of their ability to handle fear and anxiety and to communicate their feelings and concerns and to gain helpful emotional support at critical times.

Helpful hints (The Breast Cancer Handbook – I highly recommend.)

1. Ask your oncologist, oncologist nurse or hotline volunteer to recommend a support group, toll free hot line – 1-800-221-2141.
2. Support groups help you cope with your disease
3. Talk to the group leader before you join to make sure that the group is the right one for you
4. Most group leaders will suggest a trial period – an agreed upon number of sessions, before making a definite decision

LEVEL THREE – THE BODY AS A GARDEN

One metaphor from the countries of the East (India, China and Tibet) is to consider the body as a garden, and the physician as someone who attends it. I personally love the image of the human body as a garden, think of your body as a garden that needs sunlight, water, oxygen, nourishment and loving care and attention. When the garden is carefully attended, we can remove the weeds and parasites.

Always keep in mind that the body heals itself, in fact Hippocrates said that the natural healing force within each of us is the greatest force in getting well. Dr. Albert Schweitzer said each of us has a doctor within, and Thomas Edison said the medicine of the future will be natural and preventive.

Once you formally embrace this idea that the body is a garden, exercise is no longer a matter of physical exertion, it is an opportunity for bringing oxygen to the deep soil of your being.

Eating nutritious, low fat high fiber vegetarian diet with exercise or a macrobiotic diet with fish helps prevent and eliminate cancer, it is a way to nourish and fertilize the deep soil of your being.

PRACTICAL SUGGESTIONS:

Look at diet and nutrition – the cancer patient does not die from the cancer. The patient dies from malnutrition or opportunistic infection. You are not the cancer; you are more than the cancer. Cancer is a process and you are a whole person with a mind, heart and spirit. The body is temporary, while the spirit and consciousness, the soul never dies.

Adopt a plant based diet with 3-4 servings of fruit and vegetables, beans, grains, cold water fish, garlic and onions.

Eliminate all red meat and dairy products. Eliminate alcohol, refined sugar, artificial sweeteners, caffeine (use herbal teas and green tea), cigarettes and secondary smoke. You can replenish your proteins with legumes lentils, red kidney, chick beans which are high in fiber and low in fat and eat twice a week cold water fish such as salmon, mackerel, sardines or cod.

Start eating whole grains such as brown rice, spelt pasta, Jerusalem artichoke pasta and Duram wheat pasta (DiCecco brand). Buy a juicer, Juiceman Two, and start juicing fresh fruits and veggies. I own Juiceman 2 and I juice apple and carrot mixture, I also combine various cruciferous vegetables-cabbage, spinach broccoli, kale, Brussels sprouts. Cabbage has a chemical Indole Carbol 3 which helps prevent breast cancer. One can add cucumbers, parsley, celery, beets, pineapple, watermelon and cantaloupe. The combination is endless. I recommend Jay Kordich, "The Juiceman's Power of Juicing". One can get easily 3 to 4 fruits and vegetables by juicing and you can heal the body and detoxify and rejuvenate by adding the green stuff, either Green Magma Plus or Green Vibrance or Superfood (Dr Schulz) to enhance the immune system and help the skin by adding Aloe Vera liquid to the juice) avoid fried, greasy or fatty foods.

Drinks to 10 glasses of clean water to keep your body hydrated. Remember your body contains 70% water. Consider supplementing your diet with multivitamins, antioxidants and trace minerals.

Consider yourself the gift of massage at least once a week. Begin an exercise program. Start with 10 minutes and gradually increase to 30 minutes to 1 hour daily. Dancing to music is a wonderful exercise, Dr Stephen Sinatra favors dancing as an exercise.

Consider organic fruit and veggies whenever possible. For clean water consider a reverse osmosis filter or use spring water. Make sure your bowels are moving regularly eliminating toxins from your body is very important. Breathing exercises are very important to relax, get oxygen into your body and remove toxins with your out breath. Dr. Andrew Weil recommends breathing through your nose for the count four, hold it for the count of seven, and breathe out for the count of eight. Holding for the count of seven gets oxygen into your system while breathing out for a count of eight releases the waste. Dr. Weil recommends that you place your tongue against your upper teeth during the exercise. Do the exercise for four cycles.

EXPLORE THE BENEFITS OF THERAPEUTIC TOUCH

Get a hard bound journal and spend 5 to 10 minutes a day recording your thoughts, feelings and impressions. Dr. Emmett E. Miller M.D. has written a wonderful book on deep healing and he also has audiotapes on deep relaxation and visual imagery. I endorse deep relaxation and guided imagery for the cancer patient, specifically for the breast cancer patients. They can picture their body being bathed in cleansing white light or picture knights on white horses destroying the cancer cells. Some patients picture the white cells engulfing the cancer cells, completely eliminating them. It is necessary to do the deep relaxation exercises before doing the guided imagery.

I thought I would introduce you to Dr. Andrew Weil M.D., who is in charge of the Integrative Medicine Program for doctors at the University of Arizona. He is on the internet and has a program "Ask Dr. Web" and has written many books on self healing. Recently he produced a CD on meditation for optimum health with Jon Ksbat-Zinn PhD. In January 2001, Dr. Andrew Weil wrote a comprehensive plan to prevent cancer recurrence. Once Radiation, surgery and chemotherapy are finished people who have had cancer want to know, "How can I protect myself from getting cancer again"?

Cancer survivors need to pay special attention to four key areas—diet, supplements, exercise, and mind-body medicine. A whole body program – body, mind, and spirit is necessary. Enjoy fruits and vegetables. Add a rainbow mix of produce to your diet, pay particular attention to those vegetables that reduce cancer risk – such as berries, cabbage, broccoli, spinach, Brussels sprouts, cauliflower, apples and carrots.

Limit animal fats, both red meat and dairy. Try to incorporate more vegetarian dishes.

Increase your intake of Omega-3's. These cancer protective essential fatty acids are found in salmon, mackerel, sardines, halibut, cod and other cold water fish. Opt for olive oil instead of polyunsaturated vegetable oils which promote cancer. Avoid processed foods that contain hydrogenated vegetable oils. Choose foods protective against specific cancers. Eat more soy foods, soy milk (silk vanilla soy milk), tofu if you are recovering from breast cancer. Japanese women consume lots of soy products and have much less cancer.

Continue with preventing cancer recurrences. Cut back on alcohol. This advice is especially important if you have breast cancer. All authorities agree on this. Sip green tea – try to drink 3 to 4 cups daily for an optimum intake of Polyphenols that appear to reduce the risk for breast cancer. Celestial is a brand of green tea.

SUPPLEMENTS

Take antioxidants – remember that free radicals cause some 60 degenerative diseases including cancer and heart disease. And the antioxidants neutralize the free radicals and prolonging life. Each day supplement with 20000MGM vitamin C (Dr Pauling recommends much higher doses. He took 18000 MG a day; Dr. Richard Passwater recommends 2000 to 4000 mg daily for prevention in breast cancer.) 400to 800 IU of natural vitamin E,25,000 IU of Beta Carotenes, and 300 mg of Selenium to reduce the effects of carcinogens (note: this higher dose of selenium is for people who have had cancer or at increased risk.) Selenium and vitamin E work together to fight breast cancer.

Consider CO Q10 – in a few small studies, women recovering from breast cancer who took CO Q10 tended to live longer than those who did not take the supplement. Take 180 mg a day of the soft-gel form. Explore botanical remedies. You may want to try the traditional Chinese herb tonic astragalus, which is a good immune booster to take daily after treatment. Take milk thistle extract to give strength to the liver, one brand that I like is Thisilyn from Natures Waymilk; thistle repairs any liver damage.

Make room for mushrooms – to enhance immunity, look for fresh or dried Shiitake or Maitake to use in cooking. Continue with Dr. Weil-preventing cancer recurrence (Incidentally a mushroom-herb product called PC-Spes, an adaptation of a traditional Chinese remedy for cancer, appears in recent studies to benefit men with otherwise untreatable prostate cancer.)

MIND-BODY MEDICINE

Educate yourself – a good book that explores post treatment issues after cancer is after.

"Cancer: A Guide to Your New Life" by Wendy Schlessel. Get support. I suggest joining a support group for cancer survivors, either locally or online. Thanks to the groundbreaking research of David Spiegel M.D. at Stanford University and Fawzy, M.D. at UCLA with breast cancer and melanoma patients, there is little doubt that support groups can play an important role in improving survival as well as quality of life.

USE YOUR IMAGINATION

Guided imagery audiotapes made specifically for cancer survivors can help you visualize a strong, healthy and cancer-free body, or you can work with a guided imagery practitioner: for referrals contact the Academy of Guided Imagery at (800) 726-2070.

REDUCE STRESS

To improve general immune function, incorporate a relaxation technique such as breath work, meditation, self-hypnosis or yoga into your daily routine. Try Energy Medicine. Energy therapies such as therapeutic touch and Reiki may help restore harmony and shore up your defenses.

HAVE FAITH

Don't underestimate the role of your spiritual life in the Healing Process. Prayer is a powerful weapon against cancer.

EXERCISE

Exercise fights post-cancer depression and fatigue, restores immunity and helps maintain normal weight. Gradually increase physical activity: if necessary, start by walking just five minutes at a time but slowly build up to 30 minutes a day. I strongly encourage you to incorporate some of these strategies into your post-cancer life.

Dr. Andrew Weil endorses Dr. Neal Rarnard's book "Eat Right Live Longer". Dr. Weil states that Dr. Neal Barnard is one of the most responsible and authoritative voices in American medicine today.

To do your breast cells a favor, there is nothing like low fat vegetarian diet that are bodies were designed for. It easily reduces fat to around 10% of calories and provides the antioxidant-rich vegetables and fruits that keep cancer at bay. As we saw earlier soy products contain Phytoestrogens, which can mute the effects of normal estrogens, and may be part of the reason why Japanese women have such low breast cancer rates. Asian countries such as Japan have diets based on rice and vegetables with little meat and dairy products. They have had very low breast cancer rates. But as the Japanese diet has Westernized time breast cancer rate s are climbing. Women who eat meat every day are nine times the cancer risk, those who continue to base their diets on rice and vegetables have much lower cancer rates. Similar evidence comes from China; in some Chinese provinces the diet consists of rice, veggies, beans and other plant products – in these areas the cancer rate is low. As the various provinces are compared, it turns out that the more animal products in the diet, the higher the cancer rate.

Holding alcohol at arm's length helps. Even one drink a day can increase breast cancer risk 50% compared to non-drinkers.

Avoiding industrial chemicals also helps. Toxins in the air or food tend to concentrate in the breast and other fatty tissues, where they can damage the, genes. Breast cells are extremely sensitive to radiation. Current guidelines recommend routine mammography after age 50, with the proviso that the equipment be new and well-maintained to keep radiation does minimal.

In addition to improving the diet, minimizing alcohol use and avoiding radiation and chemical exposures, exercise also adds a measure of protection. Four or more hours weekly, cuts risk by 60%.

LEVEL FOUR: EMOTIONAL HEALING

An important transition takes place between Level Three and Four. So far our principal focus has been on the biological and clinical issues of cancer we looked at cancer types. Staging and treatment as well as the importance of having trust in your doctor. And the important benefits from psychological support systems. And we have considered an important new ways of looking at your body – as a garden rather than a machine and begun to explore complementary therapies.

Now the healing intention turns inward. Now the journey through cancer becomes less about cells, chemicals and diets and more about thoughts and feelings. When cancer has been detected in the breast or any other vital, organ medicine often fails to recognize that the heart is always involved. By heart I mean thoughts and feelings. If the transformation is positive, true healing can take place at every level of being. Trying to ignore or deny these feelings is fundamentally self-destructive.

After serving as physician and guide for thousands of patients and family members over many years, I can say that not one single person has ever healed from cancer without undergoing a transformation and healing of their emotional self.

Emotions have three parts: 1-thoughts, 2-feelings and 3-bodily reaction (expression). Negative thoughts trigger negative feelings which produce unpleasant body reactions such as abdominal discomfort or palpitations. Negative thoughts can trigger anger or rage which can be expressed as shouting or screaming.

There are two types of emotions – afflictive emotions which harm the body and immune system, and there are nourishing and healing emotions which heal the body and strengthen the immune system.

There is a roller coaster of emotions, fear is only the most obvious and accessible emotion associated with cancer. I've seen a full spectrum of rage, resentment, frustration, sadness, guilt, remorse doubt. Anxiety and depression occurs in up to fifty percent of cancer patients. Depression causes insomnia, early morning fatigue, difficulty concentrating, feelings of guilt, change in appetite and sex. It often presents as physical symptoms and pain. Emotions often are seen on the face. In depression the facial expression is flat and the movements are slow. Fear of death and fear of being less than a woman are very harmful emotions, but resentment is particularly a serious afflictive emotion, harmful to the body and the immune system. (T-Lymphocytes, Macrophages and natural killer cells). Resentment is a long standing feeling of wrong-doing by someone. Self-forgiveness and forgiveness are very helpful. Louise L. Hay believes that resentment is a major cause of cancer. Forgive everyone that you've felt has wronged you in your lifetime.

At the very least these emotions deserve to be acknowledged. Don't suppress your feelings. The real challenge however is working through them and finding release and freedom from them in a safe and positive way. Open up and let your emotions go. Don't bottle your feelings up. According to Lawrence Le Shan, psychologist and cancer specialist with forty years experience believes that the breast cancer patients tend to bottle up their feelings and have a problem giving and receiving love. There is very often lack of parental love-of course this is not true of every one.

Unfortunately, mainstream medicine minimized the importance of emotional work in the healing process. A major reason for this is that with exception of the psychiatrists, doctors are not trained in caring for the emotional concerns of the cancer patients and their families. In some respects, cancer is like an elephant that suddenly appears in the living room. The first order of business is to get rid of the elephant. Some get rid of everything except the elephant, some pretend the elephant isn't there. The number one priority is to address and resolve the feelings that must be dealt with or genuine healing will not occur. In fact, the damage done by cancer will still be present, it will always be present until the pain is brought out into the light of awareness and healed in the light of love. Love is the foundation of healing.

Cancer is a process that takes years to develop, but you are not the cancer, you are more than the cancer, you are the mind, heart and spirit. You are the whole person-the thoughts, feelings and spiritual self.

SOME PRACTICAL SUGGESTIONS

Here are some practical suggestions that can foster this emotional healing at any point in the journey through cancer. Remember to get a hard-bound journal and write about your experiences for at least a few minutes a day.

Remember, this is your private journal. No one else will see it without your permission, be honest with yourself. By opening up and putting your feelings – all of them – into writing will help you heal.

Ask yourself the following questions on a regular basis, and write down your answers without editing or judging them.

1. How do I feel today? What emotions have I experienced in the past twenty-four hours?
2. How do I feel about this cancer? What is it doing to my life?
3. What am I willing to give up because of this cancer?
4. What are the gifts that this cancer can bring to me and my family?
5. What can I do to make myself feel better today?

Join a support group. It is critical for you to have opportunities to share your feelings with others in a safe and healthy way. Remember your family cannot meet all your emotional needs. You can help them and yourself by finding other places for support. If you find that you are struggling with depression, anger, despair, fear guilt or resentment it is time to get some help. Consider a private therapist.

Exercise 30 minutes daily for five days a week helps relieve depression. Many breast cancer patients have benefited by a body massage weekly. Counteract fear and other afflictive, harmful emotions by deep relaxation and guided imagery (Emmett E. Miller M.D. "Deep Healing" adapted from Healing Journey-audio). The inner healer – after deep relaxation (close your eyes and breathe though your nose for count of 4, hold it for the count of 7 and breathe out for the count of 8 for 4 cycles. Make sure your tongue is placed on back of front teeth).

Use guided imagery. Picture your inner healer which can be white blood cells, engulfing and destroying the cancer cells with the help of the natural killer cells or a glowing mist of healing energy or knights on white horses or any image that works best for you. The deep relaxation and the guided imagery must be done on a daily basis.

For relaxation you could also use the relaxation response by Herbert Benson. New York: William Morrow and Co., Inc – 1975. Health is a state of physical, mental, emotional and spiritual well being.

LEVEL FIVE – THE NATURE OF THE MIND

In this level I will discuss the mind, love, belief systems and Tamoxifen. I attempt to define. The mind and love, the source of power is the one. Universal mind. God-love. a good metaphor for the universal mind is a Dynamo. The Dynamo or A/C generator is the power that runs all the electricity in the house.

The mind has two aspects, a double thread: The objective, conscious mind in the material world which strives for a strong ego and self-esteem and the subjective, invisible subconscious mind that embraces peace and stillness without the ego. The conscious mind tells the subconscious what to do, and the SUBCONSCIIOUS IS like a puppy dog and carries out the orders without question.

In this segment I will introduce you to Louise L. Hay who had a dysfunctional life, raped as a child, divorced several times, developed terminal cancer and cured herself. She went on to become internationally famous healing others. Her message is simple: Love yourself just as you are and approve of yourself. In the pages that follow I will explain the exercises that she uses and recommends that you use on a daily basis.

The essence of our being is love and the foundation for healing is love. A powerful high intensity energy, we are spiritual beings with human experiences and it is important to stay connected to the source, the universal mind, God – Love. When we separate from the source problems arise. Dr. Wayne Dwyer believes that there is a spiritual solution to every problem and has written a book on this topic.

Louise L. Hay ends each session with the following:

In the infinity of life where I am now, all is perfect, whole and complete. All is well in my life.

RESS, RELAXATION AND VISUAL IMAGERY

Stress is a force with psychological and physiological stressors causing bodily damage. The external stressors can be viruses, infection or shock while the internal stressors can be fear, anxiety and depression. Threat of impending danger is a major stressor and the most severe stress is death of a spouse, divorce, severe illness and death of a family member. The most amazing fact is that the reaction to stress is the same regardless of the nature of the stressor.

There is always an imbalance of the autonomic nervous system and an activation of the sympathetic nervous system preparing the person for fight or flight. There is an increase in blood pressure, pulse, blood sugar, muscle spasm, breathing and oxygen. The acute stress is due to Adrenalin while chronic stress is due to Cortisol. Stress is a risk factor for heart disease, cancer and can make diabetes worse. Many of the risk factors for cancer and heart disease are similar (elevation of cholesterol, smoking, hypertension, inactivity, obesity). Stress is a risk factors for cancer and heart disease. Stress can weaken the immune system and contribute to the development of cancer. Stress can be good or bad, Hans Selye, the father of stress is concerned about the bad stress leading to distress and depression.

The key to stress management is how we handle stress. Stress can be handled by deep relaxation and visual imagery. The Nervous system doesn't know the difference from that which is real from that which is in the room of your mind. The feeling is the same. Whatever you picture and believe, you can achieve. It is important to use the five senses when doing visual imagery. Use sight (color), feelings, smell, sound and taste.

Shakespeare wrote "nothing is good or bad, but thinking makes it so". Thoughts must be applied with care in the journey through cancer. I don't intend that cancer is caused by "wrong" thoughts or that it can be cured by "right" thoughts and I don't want to suggest that getting cancer is "good". However the experience of cancer is a subjective one. Our thoughts profoundly affect our experiences in the real world.

What is our mind? Our mind is subjective, invisible and is a source of energy. The mind is a function of the brain. The brain is matter and weighs three pounds and we can hold it in our hands, while the mind is invisible and we cannot hold it in our hands. The mind influences the body and the body influences the mind. They work together. The thoughts are electrical energy and create our future. We can change our thoughts and we can only have one thought at a time. The amazing fact is that we have control of our mind and have the choice to use it any way we want.

The source of power is the universal mind, which is everywhere and represents love, God and nature, the universal mind is like a Dynamo and runs everything just like the generators that give us electricity to run our appliances, TV, computer, refrigerator, stove etc. The universal mind in the human takes on two aspects, the objective mind in the material world and the "subjective mind" sometimes called the subconscious. The objective mind is analytical while the subconscious is automatic, spontaneous and creative. It is the doer. It carries whatever the "conscious mind" suggests. When man thinks he is drawing power from the infinite "voltage" of the universal mind. The objective mind is not the doer, the action takes place in the "subconscious".

The spirit is the primary cause and has a positive polarity and is attracted to the objective mind, which has a negative polarity. Energy is interchangeable with matter. The spirit is energy that never dies while the body is temporary and is impermanent like everything on earth. The spirit is the primary cause and the effect is matter, the mind is the builder and is responsible for transferring thought energy to thought form (matter). Look around and everything that you see, the TV, stove, vacuum cleaner, and chair was all started in somebody's mind as a thought. There are certain things that man is unable to create. Man cannot make a tree, an ocean a robin.

The interesting fact is our thoughts; feelings and spirit are all energy. Our thoughts are electrical energy and our feelings are chemical energy. Positive thoughts, self love and joy produce good feelings while negative thoughts anger, hatred, guilt, self criticism, resentment produce unpleasant feelings. Resentment eats away at our bodies and can even contribute to cancer, while forgiveness of self and others dissolves the resentment. A healthy attitude, self love makes for physiological and psychological balance, wholeness and healing,

The patients with an unhealthy attitude and lifestyle react with feelings of powerlessness, loneliness and deprivation. The result is emotional and physiologic stress and disease (the stress is aggravated by genetic predisposition and environment). Elliott S. Dacher, M.D.

developed the new mind/body healing program. The program is based on psychoneuroimmunology-mind, nervous system and immunology.

According to Dr. Dacher, the mind works in two ways, mind-talk and mindfulness. Mind talk is predominant and automatic and is expressed by thoughts, feelings, sensations and images. Mind talk directs our day to day lives. We can shut off our automatic mind and switch to mindfulness. Mindfulness is attention, concentration and meditation. It is non—judgmental, moment to moment awareness.

Our thoughts move so quickly that we experience them as a continuous stream. A diagnosis of cancer has an instant and extremely powerful effect on the thinking process. Now there are variations on a single theme: "Why did I get cancer? Where can I get the best treatment? I'm terrified what is going to happen to me?" The mind is sometimes described as a monkey, jumping from tree to tree, never stopping in normal life. The "monkey mind" jumps from thought to thought, covering a wide range of subjects.

I endorse the philosophy of Louise L. Hay as presented in her book "You Can Heal Your Life" the bottom line for everyone is I'm not good enough". Resentment, criticism and guilt are the most damaging patterns. In my opinion there are no justified resentments. Dissolve resentment with forgiveness of self and others. It is very harmful to carry around daily hatred for real or imaginary wrong-doings. Persistent hatred and blame damages the body and weakens the immune system. According to Louse, releasing resentment will dissolve even cancer. When we really love ourselves, everything in life works. We must release the past and forgive everyone (the course in miracles stresses forgiveness).

We must be willing to begin to learn to love ourselves. Self-approval and self acceptance in the now is the key to positive changes. We create every so-called "illness" in our body.

We are each 100% responsible for all of our experiences. If we take complete responsibility we can't blame anyone. When we blame we give away our power. Replace hatred with love. Fear cannot exist in the presence of love.

One of the best exercises for self-image is the mirror exercise (Louise Hay) look at yourself in the mirror and say your name and repeat, "I love myself just the way I am", do this every morning for 30 days and during the day as often as possible. Say "I approve of myself" your inner self will accept this and carry it out. Say it, believe it, achieve it. Louise L Hay is a bestselling author who had vaginal cancer and healed herself. Louise Hay's key message is if we are willing to do the mental work, almost anything can be healed". She had terminal cancer and cured herself. As a metaphysical counselor, she devotes her life to assisting others in removing the blocks that keep them from robust health.

Louise hay uses the mirror exercise every day, before lunch she likes to go to the mirror and do some affirmations out loud and they go something like this:

Louise, you are wonderful and I love you. This is one of the best days of my life. Everything is working out for your highest good whatever you need to know is revealed for you. Whatever you need comes to you. All is well.

I have done this exercise myself for thirty days and I felt great.

Another exercise is excellent for relationships and attracting love. Get a pad and write the following:

I love myself therefore . . . . I am able to love others and God more passionately.
I love myself therefore . . . . I behave and think in a loving way to all people for I know that which I give out returns to me multiplied.
I love myself therefore I am willing to fight hard, accept the challenge and heal the cancer. For I know that the body heals itself and that there are no incurable diseases.
I love myself therefore I forgive and totally release the past and all past experiences and I am free.
I love myself therefore; I am willing to dissolve all anger hatred and resentments.
I love myself therefore, I am willing to change for I know that I am a spiritual being with human experiences and in the infinity of life where I am, all is perfect, whole and complete, All is well in my world.
I love myself therefore; I take loving care of my body. I lovingly feed it nourishing foods and beverages. I lovingly groom it and dress it and my body lovingly responds with vibrant health and energy.

In this exercise you can add whatever you want to the therefore. Ask yourself what you want, take action watch what you are getting and make the necessary changes to get what you want. Knowledge is good, but knowledge without action is useless. In other words, if you keep doing the same thing, you keep getting the same results. The ancestor of all action is a thought and the father of action is a decision.

What is love? According to Jose Silva, love is the opposite of hate. Love is a powerful, higher energy than hate which is a weaker lower energy. According to Erich Fromm love is an art requiring concentration patience, self-discipline and practice. Quote from Kabil Gibran: "The chemist who can extract from his heart's elements compassion, respect, longing, patience, regret, surprise and forgiveness and compound them into one can create that atom which is called love."

My definition of love is as follows: Love is a giving of positive powerful higher energy to yourself and to the core of another being (the spirit) so as to fully nourish it. Love is what you experience after true forgiveness. "Love" in Aramaic, is a condition in the mind that each individual is responsible for maintaining. It is the fuel that empowers the human mind to function correctly. The human mind can't function correctly when we are angry, hostile, afraid or resentful.

BELIEFS

We've seen how thoughts can have a life of their own particularly under the stressful conditions encountered in the diagnosis of cancer. Beliefs are a sense of certainty; they involve a higher level of commitment than our thoughts. Beliefs about cancer are more deeply ingrained and slower to change. Beliefs most often originate in childhood. Parents are by far the most important. If parents told you over and over again: "men don't cry", "watch what you say", and "you can't trust anyone". These unconscious beliefs have an effect on your relationships. Beliefs can also come from events in your life and relationship with teachers and institutions. In dealing with patients' beliefs I have found that it is much more useful to ask questions than to make directive statements.

1) What are your empowering beliefs about cancer? My body has the ability to heal itself of cancer; cancer will be a challenge, but it won't destroy me. I will win this battle, because I want to live and enjoy life.

What are my disempowering beliefs about cancer? Cancer is a deadly process; cancer will wreck my life.

2) What are my empowering beliefs about doctors? Doctor's are knowledgeable and some of them do care. Doctors are trustworthy and some of them tell the truth. What are my disempowering beliefs about doctors? Doctors are greedy. Doctors are untrustworthy; doctors don't really tell the truth. Doctors are knowledgeable, but uncaring.

3) What are your disempowering beliefs about cancer? I got cancer because I smoked. Because I ate bad food and had a unhealthy lifestyle. I got cancer because I had an unhealthy attitude. Because I inherited bad genes from my parents.

4) What are my disempowering beliefs about chemotherapy? Chemotherapy is poison and will not save my life. Chemotherapy will destroy my immune system. Chemotherapy is only effective in three percent of cancer patients. Chemotherapy will make me sick with nausea and vomiting etc. What are my empowering beliefs about chemotherapy? Chemotherapy will save my life. Chemotherapy will help me.

5) What are your beliefs and expectations about what will happen to you? I will probably die. I don't know what will happen to me.

6) What are your empowering beliefs about God? I believe that there is a supreme being called God who is kind and good. I believe that god is all loving.

7) What are your beliefs about spirituality? I believe that we are spiritual beings with human experiences. Spirituality is important to me.

Make a list of your empowering and disempowering beliefs about cancer, God, spirituality and about death and life after death.

For example—do you believe that there is life after death and that our spirit (energy) and soul (consciousness) never die? We just pass over and the body is temporary. Or do you believe that nothing exists beyond death.

If we have an empowering belief and a healthy attitude we will tap into our potential, and increase our potential, then action will insure an excellent result.

What are your empowering beliefs about Tamoxifen?

1) I believe that Tamoxifen is anti-estrogenic and could improve my chances of having a recurrence and live a long and healthy life.
2) I could improve my chances of avoiding heart disease and osteoporosis.
3) I could gain the knowledge that I was getting the benefit of everything that medical science has to offer me right now.

What are your disempowering beliefs about Tamoxifen? Do you believe:

1) It has many side effects, such as forming blood clots
2) It is an unnatural substance
3) It will decrease my sex drive
4) It will make me have hot flashes
5) It will increase my risk of uterine cancer

Nolvadex (Tamoxifen)

Tamoxifen is an anticancer drug. It may be given to treat breast cancer. It also has proved effective when cancer has spread to other parts of the body. It is most effective in stopping the kind of breast cancer that thrives on estrogen. Most important fact about this drug is Women taking Tamoxifen should have routine GYN exams and report any abnormal vaginal bleeding, vaginal discharge or pelvic pain. Take the drug as prescribed. It may be necessary to take the drug for several years. Side effects from Tamoxifen are usually mild. More common side effects are hot flashes, nausea and vomiting. Rare side effects may include blood clots or visual disturbances. Special warning – if you have visual disturbances while taking Tamoxifen, notify your doctor immediately.

The daily dosage ranges from 20 to 40 Mg day. If you are taking more than 20 Mg, your doctor will have you divide the total into two smaller doses taken in the morning and evening. Our experience of events is not only influenced by our thoughts, beliefs, but by what you focus on. The meaning we give to cancer and what we focus on influences the outcome. The patients who have empowering beliefs and give positive meanings and focus on the positive aspects do better. Those who believe in a higher power and pray; those who accept cancer as a challenge and are determined to defeat it with all possible resources often end up victorious. Remember we can change our feelings by what we focus on, by our beliefs by the questions we ask and by our words.

When I have a challenge, I ask what I want. Not what I don't want. Take action, watch what I am getting and keep changing until I get what I want. In your case, ask what do you want? Do you want to accept the challenge to fight and heal the cancer? You have the potential to heal this cancer. Another important question is why do you want to live? Find as many reasons as possible for wanting to live. This will motivate you, if you have enough whys then the how is easier.

After you have made a commuted decision, take action. The father of all action is a committed decision, then watch what you are getting (want it to happen, expect it to happen, watch it happen), then keep changing until you get the desired result.

Presently, you need to improve the immune system (white cells) and manage stress, what should you do immediately? I would purchase a juicer (The Juiceman II by Jay Kordich). I have been juicing for years and own the Juiceman II by Jay Kordich. By the way Jay Kordich had cancer when he was young and went to Max Gerson's clinic and started juicing with apples and carrots and healed his cancer. Today he is over age 70. To order your Juiceman II for free info call—1-800-233-9054. Juicing helps both the immune system and stress.

Neuroscientists (Candice Pert—Psychoneuroimmunology) have shown that thoughts, feelings and beliefs influence the immune system. The immune system will benefit from a positive, healthy mental attitude, juicing, diet, exercise and relaxation techniques, deep relaxation and guided imagery (Picture the cancer cells being destroyed by cleansing white light and white cells engulfing the cancer cells)

LEVEL SIX – LIFE ASSESSMENT

This program is an invitation to understand, explore and reconnect with your purposes of your life. We all want pleasure and avoid pain. We automatically go towards pleasure, and away from pain. Our true nature is to be happy, and have peace of mind and experience love and joy. Learn how to use pain and pleasure, and don't let pain and pleasure use you. You can consciously create your own circumstances.

We are unique and experience pleasure differently. Make a list of your pleasures in life. For example, some experience pleasure by exercising, dancing, listening to music, traveling, going to art museums, taking photos, or helping others get what they want. Some get pleasure out of learning and growing.

The words that cause pain and overwhelming fear are "I'm sorry, but you have cancer" "Am I going to die"? What does my future have in store for me? Usually all cancer patients initially have some kind of physical, mental, emotional and spiritual pain.

Down deep everyone with cancer wants to think and feel better. How? We can change the way we think and feel. We can do this by changing what we focus on, our body language, words, self-talk and the questions we ask. The ancestor of all action is our thoughts. Our thoughts create our future. Every though has a feeling. Good loving thoughts produce pleasant feelings.

We don't die from cancer. Cancer is a process. And we are not the cancer. We are more than the cancer. We are the whole person, heart, mind and spirit. There is overwhelming evidence that the spirit and soul don't die. We are spiritual beings with human experiences, and are connected to god. Our essence is love and joy.

Raymond Moody M.D. offers astonishing proof of a life after physical death, his book "Life After Life" is a classic another wonderful book "We Don't Die" about the experiences of George Anderson and his spiritual communications. "I Want You To Understand That

Life Is Everlasting, and Everything That Happens In Your Life Has a Purpose"

Level six of this program describes a process for identifying the means and purpose of life. Clarifying specific goals for the coming year and considering how you wish to be remembered after you are gone.

There are three very important reasons why finding clear and coherent answers to these questions is so important on the journey through cancer. First: cancer often brings about difficult and challenging times. It is important to know why you want to live and have a clear and compelling motivation for fighting on. You must believe and have the courage to fight to heal and cure this cancer. You are to focus on reasons for living. I personally believe that ten years means a cure, not 5 years. I have seen patients with a fighting spirit with breast cancer go into a complete remission. Some patients live years longer than expected, while many factors influence the outcome, it is clear that the patients benefited from well-defined and compelling reasons for living. Fredric Nietzsche wrote, "He who has an important enough why can bear almost anyhow."

We have seen cancer challenges patients and family members go through. Cancer patients simply cannot afford unfulfilling or destructive thoughts, activities and relationships. Many people finally stop smoking, drinking, change their diet and start exercising.

Third: some people will discover that they don't want to fight their disease. Patients may feel for whatever reason they are unwilling to undergo Surgery, radiation or chemotherapy, or even alternative or complementary approaches to healing.

THE LIFE—ASSESSMENT PROCESS

We have covered many important issues in the preceding pages, to help patients address these issues; I ask them to begin responding in writing to some basic questions.

What is the meaning and purpose of your life?
What are your most important goals for the next year?
How do you want to be remembered after you are gone?

What is the meaning and purpose of your life?

If I may use myself as an example I would say that the purpose of my life is to know and celebrate my true self – the timeless, eternal essence of God, of spirit and of all beings and to be a powerful presence of love, joy, wisdom, compassion, awareness, and truth for myself and others. It has been humorously said, "At the end of your life, God will not ask you, 'why didn't you spend more time at the office?' The important questions are: Did I know my true self? Did I live the highest values? Did I live life to the fullest? Most importantly, Did I love myself as well as others – Did I help others get what they want?

It is clear to me that the ultimate purpose of this new paradigm of medicine is to assist all beings to experience unbounded love and joy and to know that this is the essence of who we are.

My mission however, is to create a new paradigm of medicine that promotes awareness, healing and transformation at the deepest levels of body, mind, heart and spirit of all beings.

When I met Dr. Geffen M.D., I gave him my definition of love. Love is the giving of powerful positive energy to oneself and to the core of somebody else's being–the spirit, so as to nourish it. Loving kindness from my heart to yours.

My purpose in life is to be happy, have peace of mind and be of service to others and to learn and grow and most of all to love myself, love God and love others. To me, happiness is thinking positive, constructive thoughts most of the time.

Beverly, a breast cancer patient, after closing her eyes and going deeply into her heart wrote:

"The purpose of my life is to experience abundant love, joy and peace in my heart and to experience physical, mental, emotional and spiritual health and freedom and to share this with others."

What are your most important goals for the next year?

When you set a goal, you've commit feed to "Cani". You have acknowledged. ("Cani" means constant, never-ending improvement).

The need that all human beings have for constant, never-ending improvement and goals should be specific and require a time frame. Consider the following categories for the next year: physically, mentally, emotionally, spiritually, relationships, attractiveness socially, career and financially.

1. To become healthy strong and energetic
2. Not to worry or be fearful – to have a healthy, positive attitude
3. To take one day at a time and find joy every day
4. Have a family reunion and visit my children and grandchildren
5. Take time each day to read the bible and pray
6. Stop looking like a cancer patient and be more at peace with life
7. Find more courage and face my cancer as a challenge rather than an obstacle
8. Take an interest in cooking and having friends for dinner

How do you want to be remembered?

A third part of the life-assessment process has to do with acknowledging the fact that some time in the future we are all destined to die. This is true regardless of our circumstances in life.

"How do you want to be remembered'?" When done properly and with sensitivity, helping patients and family members explore this question in a loving and supportive way can yield insights and breakthroughs that are moving, profound and important.

Kate Seymour a cancer patient gave her list. Here it is:

How and what I want to be remembered for in my life.

1. Someone who cared deeply for family
2. A loving wife, a good listener, someone with a good sense of humor
3. A caring mother and friend
4. A faithful servant of God
5. Someone who was nonjudgmental and sensitive to others' needs
6. Someone who had courage in the face of adversity

Stress can cause a chemical imbalance in the nervous system. Stress means different things to different people. Stress is a demand on you to adjust. To accept. To change. Those demands are stressors, as we mentioned before. Irrational thoughts produce irrational feelings, if thoughts of what has happened in the past or of what is happening now keep flashing into your mind or if you keep dwelling into the past, say out loud "Stop". After about a week of saying "Stop" out loud you will be able to think stop and the word "Stop" becomes a conditioned reflex.

The opposite of anxiety is relaxation. When you are relaxed you can't feel tension. Dr. Herman M. Zeidman M.D., M.S. (Psch) is a personal friend and he has developed a wonderful one minute relaxation exercise. You can do it anywhere and anytime. This relaxation exercise takes 1 minute to do, but you must do it six times a day for the first week. It will counteract anxiety. Practice makes perfect. Memorize these directions and follow them exactly.

Sit in a comfortable chair with your feet flat on the floor, and hands on your lap. There are five steps:

Step1 – Touch the tips of your right thumb and right index finger together making a circle. After a week it will become a conditioned reflex.

Step 2 – Close your eyes gently and take three deep breaths slowly relaxing your shoulders during each exhalation.

Steps 3 – Think of the beach, if you have another favorite place it's OK to visualize that place instead and now in the same order visualize A – The warmth of the sun, B – The color of the water. Rotating your senses like this helps you relax. C – The smell of the fresh air. D – The sound of the surf.

Step 4 – Now, with your eyes still closed, picture a blackboard with three words on it: Confident – Calm – Relaxed.

Steps 5 – Now say to yourself, "Now I am going to count up to three to come out of this relaxed state, feeling alert and refreshed" slowly count to three and open your eyes.

You will find each time you do this one minute relaxation exercise, your feeling of self-confidence and self esteem will strengthen without a feeling of self-value, your anxieties can not be controlled. You must memorize the entire exercise. Steps one, two and five are easy to memorize. Steps three and four are a little more complicated.

STRESS, RELAXATION AND VISUAL IMAGERY

Stress is a force with psychological and physiological stressors causing bodily damage. The external stressors can be viruses, infection shock while the internal stressors can be fear, anxiety and depression. Threat of impending danger is a major stressor and the most severe stress is death of a spouse, divorce, severe illness and death of a family member. The most amazing fact is that the reaction to stress is the same regardless of the nature of the stressor. There is always an imbalance of the autonomic nervous system and an activation of the sympathetic nervous system preparing the person for fight or flight. There is an increase in blood pressure, pulse, blood sugar, muscle spasm, breathing and oxygen. The acute stress is due to adrenalin while chronic stress is due to cortisol. Stress is a risk factor for heart disease, cancer and can make diabetes worse. Many of the risk factors for cancer and heart disease are similar. Elevation of cholesterol, smoking, hypertension, inactivity, obesity, stress is risk factors for cancer and heart disease. Stress can weaken the immune system and contribute to the development of cancer. Stress can be good or bad. Hans Selye, the father of stress, is concerned about the bad stress leading to distress and depression. The key to stress management is how we handle stress. Stress can be handled by deep relaxation and visual imagery. The nervous system doesn't't know the difference between that which is real from that which is in the room of your mind. The feeling is the same. Whatever you picture and believe, you can achieve, it is important to use the five senses when doing visual imagery. Use sight (color), feelings, smell sound and taste.

Visual imagery – The image of the ocean, beach and sunrise. Begin by sitting in a comfortable chair and place both feet on ground and both hands on your lap. Close your eyes and take two deep breaths through your nose. Now, count from 5 to 1 with each count feel more and more relaxed. (use diaphragmatic breathing-let the abdomen rise with each inhalation and go down with each exhalation, now take a deep breath through your nose, and hold it slightly and with the out breath say 5 and deeply relax another deep breath through your nose and hold it slightly and with the out breath say 4 and deeply relax, another deep breath through your nose, hold it slightly and with the out breath say 3 and deeply relax, another deep breath through your nose and hold it slightly, and with the out breath say 2, twice as relaxed now, take a deep breath through your nose and hold it slightly for a few seconds and with the out breath say one, the bottom of relaxation, the cellar of relaxation. deeply relaxed.

Now that you are deeply relaxed, in the room of your mind picture the sun rising behind a cloud, see an orange, red ball moving higher, the color changes to golden yellow and then white, feel the warmth of the sun, smell the fresh air, hear the sound of the waves, and see the ebb and flow of the waves. As the waves move out and in you feel more and more relaxed and finally you can even taste the salt water.

Now count from 1 to 3 with each count feel more and more awake and alert. Move around look at your watch, feel wonderfully refreshed. In this exercise you have used the 5 senses and your imagination.

The nervous system does not know the difference between what is real and what is in the room of your mind. This exercise I have developed and use frequently to relax. It is very important to follow the sensory sequence: Color, feeling of warmth, smell, sound, vision of the waves going in and out, and finally the taste.

STRESS AND RELAXATION

"Stress is the non-specific response of the body to any demand". It is manifested first by an alarm reaction, followed by a stage of resistance during which increased defenses to the stressor occur and finally a stage of exhaustion resulting in disease, fatigue or death. This is called the "general adaptation syndrome"—Hans Selye.

Stress is a non-specific reaction to a perceived demand put upon the body; the most important factor is how you perceive the stress.

Stress can be good or bad, but if you perceive the stress as threat, then the flight-fight reaction is activated. For example, public speaking is the number #1 fear for most people, but for some it is enjoyable and giving a speech is fun. The threat can be real or imaginary. Mark Twain once said, "I'm an old man and have known a great many troubles, most of which never happened."

Stress can be acute, chronic or post-traumatic stress syndrome, most stress is acute with the release of adrenalin, activating the flight-fight reaction, chronic stress releases cortisol which is responsible for much disease and post-traumatic distress common in the Vietnam war, characterized by flash backs and night-mares.

Stress is an imbalance of the involuntary, autonomic nervous system. The involuntary nervous system is responsible for the heart rate breathing and glandular secretion and is separate from the central nervous system which we have control. The autonomic nervous system is divided into the sympathetic, which releases energy and the parasympathetic nervous system which conserves and restores energy. In stress, there is an activation of the sympathetic nervous system with release of adrenalin from the adrenal gland, arousing the individual for fight or flight. There is a unified reaction resulting in elevation of blood pressure, increase in heart rate, elevation of blood sugar, increase in blood clotting, muscular tension and spasm of neck and shoulder muscles. Rapid, shallow, irregular breathing, increase in oxygenation, the increase in glucose and oxygen are needed by the brain. The brain is nourished by sugar and oxygen. So stress can cause hypertension, irregular heart rhythms, heart attacks, stroke, headache, arthritis and muscular-skeletal disorders.

For example, most heart attacks occur on Monday morning around 9 AM for those going to a job they hate. There are two important questions to ask "Do I enjoy my job"? and am I happy with my life"? In prehistoric times, the cave man reacted to stress by fighting animals, or running away. In modern society we usually don't punch people in the nose or run and hide, we bottle up the energy internally causing bodily reaction and disease.

The stressors can be external, physical such as hot, cold, infection, shock, pain or internal, mental such as anger, fear, anxiety, depression or resentment. The major causes of stress are death of a spouse, divorce, severe illness, and illness in the family, death of family member, financial loss, death or illness of a friend.

There are three structures in the brain that play a big part in stress: The hypothalamus, pituitary gland and the adrenal. The hypothalamus releases the cortical releasing factor which stimulates the pituitary gland to release the adrenocorticotropic hormone that stimulates the adrenal to release adrenalin.

Chronic stress and lack of balance contribute to illness. Likewise, relaxation, positive methods of coping with stress and restoration of balance lead to health by becoming actively involved in self-healing one shifts from the feelings of helplessness and hopelessness that have been shown to increase depression and the risk of death to a sense of control.

The best way to handle stress is by using relaxation techniques. There are numerous healing modalities such as:

1. The Relaxing Breath by Dr. Weil
2. The Relaxation Response developed By Herbert Benson M.D.
3. Deep relaxation and guided visual imagery (ideal for cancer patients)
4. Meditation-Non-Judgmental Moment to Moment Awareness – Jon-Kabbat Zinn
5. Self-hypnosis by Dr. Alosi
6. Prayer
7. Yoga
8. Massage
9. Humor

The important message that follows is that stress, the response to the demand put upon the body and mind, fear of divorce, fear of illness, fear of death of loved ones, inhibits the immune system causing an under reaction and cancer, breathing exercises and deep relaxation with guided imagery enhances and strengthens the immune system (white blood cells, T-lymphocytes, macrophages and killer cells). Now, we are concentrating on stress management and the immune system. As previously discussed, there are additional ways to enhance the immune system. Diet, nutrition (detoxification, juicing with greens) a healthy attitude and life style, self-regulation and exercise will make the immune system stronger and result in balance, wholeness and healing.

Herbs and nutritional supplements will also enhance the immune system. The major herbs are garlic, Echinacea, Astragulus and Aloe Vera. The major supplements are vitamin C, E, Beta carotene, Zinc, Selenium and CO Enzyme-Q 10.

SELF-HYPNOSIS AND BREAST CANCER

All hypnosis is self hypnosis. You give suggestions to yourself. Self-hypnosis uses hyper-suggestibility. The mind – consciousness has three levels: Conscious, unconscious and subconscious.

The conscious mind is only analytical and compares but does not do anything. The unconscious mind is automatic such as breathing and heart beat. It is protective. The subconscious mind is where all the action is. The subconscious mind harbors all our experiences, habits and beliefs. The subconscious mind is automatic, spontaneous, creative and is the doer.

I send positive thoughts, feelings, memories and pictures to my subconscious mind.

> I want to feel secure, fair and worthy.
> When I feel secure, I knock out fear.
> When I relax, I knock out fear.
> When I feel that life is fair,
> I knock out anger.
> When I feel worthy,
> I knock out unworthiness

According to Louise Hay, she only works on feelings of unworthiness. I want to feel worthy. When I feel worthy, fair and secure I turn on my protective genes that heal the breast cancer. When I relax, I give positive suggestions via self-hypnosis to analyze the situation and the result is healing.

Oncogenes cause breast cancer.

The P53 protective genes heal breast cancer.

Positive emotions like love, joy and peace heal the cancer and turn on the protective genes. A healthy diet with fruits, vegetables, grains beans and nuts heal. A healthy life style, exercise, elimination of alcohol and smoking, low fat diet turn on the protective genes. Nutrition plays a big part in healing of the breast cancer (Dr Charles Simeone). Some of the material comes from Dr Cal Banyan's course on the "7th Path of Self Hypnosis, Language of Feelings."

The next 3 pages will discuss breathing, immune system and deep relaxation with guided imagery.

I have introduced you to the one minute relaxation exercise and the beach exercise using visual imagery. Now, I would like to teach you a simple yoga-derived relaxing breath exercise which is the standard at the University of Arizona under Dr. Weil. In this exercise you will observe your breath, make your breathing deep, slow and regular instead of shallow, rapid and irregular. When you relax your breathing will become, silent, deep, slow and regular.

Breathe abdominally, place your hand on your belly and when you inhale your abdomen will rise and when you exhale your belly will move back in. Now, on with the exercise:

1. Sit or lie comfortably with your back straight and place your tongue between your teeth and palate. (Yoga position) keep your tongue there for the entire exercise. Close your eyes.
2. Exhale completely through the mouth, making an audible whoosh sound
3. Close your mouth lightly, inhale through your nose quietly to the count of four.
4. Hold it for the count of seven (allows oxygen into your system)
5. Exhale audibly through your mouth to the count of eight. If you have difficulty exhaling with your tongue in place, try pursing your lips (instead of my tongue between my teeth and palate, I prefer to place my thumb and index finger together forming an 0 for the duration of the exercise) the exhalation releases co2 and waste products.
6. 6-repeat steps 3 through 5 three more times for a total of four cycles. Breathe normally and observe how your body feels. This

exercise produces a pleasant state which feels better with regular practice.

Do this exercise for 5 minutes morning an evening before bedtime. After one month increase the cycles to 8. The key to this exercise is keeping the ratio 4-7-8. I find this exercise helps me fall asleep and get back to sleep if I wake up during the night. Use this exercise where you are anxious, angry, upset or when you are experiencing discomfort.

This exercise does three things, it causes relaxation, increases oxygen into your system and gets rid of waste products during the out breath (the cancer patient benefits from increased oxygenation).

The next exercise is the relaxation response by Herbert Benson. This exercise uses a mantra or special sound, such as OM or one. It is referred to as TM or transcendental meditation. This is a very easy exercise.

Sit in a comfortable chair, straight back with hands on your lap and both feet on the floor. Close your eyes and take. In a deep breath, you can hold it slightly. Exhale and say OM with each out breath. I find this very relaxing.

Now take another deep breath and repeat this over and over, saying OM with each out breath. Do this for 15 minutes in the morning and evening. The heart rate slows and the breathing becomes deep, slow and regular.

Deep relaxation and guided visual imagery is one of the most important exercises for the cancer patient. It is a good idea to have some understanding of the immune system before discussing the technique; the immune system is a surveillance system, a defensive system that is on guard for foreign invaders like bacteria, viruses and cancer cells, in the blood stream. There are white blood cells, T-Lymphocytes, Macrophages, natural killer cells and antibodies. These cells are intelligent and have a mind of their own and talk to each other. When a cancer cell presents itself the T-Lymphocyte lets the Macrophages know about it and these cells engulf the cancer cells and also communicate information to the natural killer cells. The immune system functions as a second brain and is so intelligent that it is capable of allowing a remission to take place; T-Lymphocytes originate in the thymus gland which is under the breast bone, while the antibodies come from the bone marrow. The macrophages engulf the cancer cells and destroy them and the killer cells also destroy cancer cells. When the body is under stress, production of the natural "killer" cells, called T-Lymphocytes and Macrophages, seems to be inhibited, the inhibition probably occurs because of excess cortisol. The hormone, cortisol is produced because of chronic stress. This may be the connection between stress and the development of cancer.

Pschoneuroimmunology is the new mind-body medicine, which states that the mind, nervous system and the immune system are all connected, the brain (hypothalamus-structure in the mid brain) relays an informational substance to the cells and genes of the lymphocytes, the immune cells are mobile and move with lightning speed through the blood stream (milliseconds), so there is rapid communication between the brain and the immune system and vice versa.

When there is an under-reaction of the immune system internally, tumor and cancer results. If the under reaction is external then a cold or virus may present itself. Thoughts, feelings and beliefs influence the immune system. Depression, anger, sadness and fear weaken the immune system, while love, joy and peace strengthen the immune system. Fear interferes with performance and results in inhibition of the natural "killer cells", love neutralizes fear.

In addition to stress, toxins from air, food and water can damage the immune system. The toxins cause free radicals which can break through the cell membranes and get into the DNA and cause mutations and cancer. So it is imperative that you have a healthy attitude and life style. The bottom line is a healthy diet, fruits, veggies, beans, grains, nuts, mainly vegetarian with cold water fish, low fat, nutritional supplements, herbs and deep relaxation techniques preferably with visual imagery.

Focus on the ways your health is affected by your beliefs and feelings. Your beliefs, sense of certainty guide your life. It is important for you to believe that you have an inner healer and that you can heal yourself and take responsibility for your healing. Hippocrates said that the body heals itself and Dr. Albert Schweitzer said that we have a physician within us. Deep healing depends on deep relaxation and guided visual imagery of ideal health. Imagine traveling through your body and see areas that you want to heal. You might get good results from images of healing, cleansing white light destroying the invaders such as cancer cells or viruses, or knights on white horses or superheroes swooping down to knock out and annihilate all infection or cancer cells.

After going into a deeply relaxed state using some of the previous relaxation exercises, then visualize this exercise called the "inner healer". Your inner healer may be white blood cells, an army of doctors or nurses knights on white horses, a glowing mist of healing energy or whatever image works for you. Watch the process as if you are watching a movie or television program see, hear and feel the cleansing, healing process. With each breath your body is sending more healing energy to the area.

That you are imagining. Picture your body as whole, healthy, strong and vital. You see your inner healer finish this marvelous healing work, see yourself as already healed. You are in control you are no longer helpless or hopeless, you see yourself in control, masterful confronting any situation with success, confidence and a winning way.

Thousands of people have greatly benefited from this healing exercise, healing gradually over a period of time. Make this exercise a regular part of your daily life and you will be surprised by the results. An excellent resource-read the book getting well again by Carl Simonton M.D. In 1977 Emmett F. Miller M.D. co-founded the cancer support and education center in Menlo Park, CA. Much of their work has to do with the links between disease and our ability to express ourselves. Some of the most important aspects of what cancer patients learn is to be more assertive, to feel comfortable with being who they are and to give themselves permission to live fully,

The section we are on now is mainly Stress Management and Relaxation Techniques which have spiritual value. This next section is on mindfulness meditation. These ideas come mainly from Dr. Deepak Chopra. Mindfulness meditation is really non-judgmental moment to moment awareness. It involves just being non-doing and breathing. You are a silent observer watching your thoughts, feelings, sensations as they come and go. Always returning to your breathing.

It is a mind—body connection. Your thoughts represent the mind while the breathing represents the body. I lecture to various groups in Florida and recently took part in a group discussion on nature of thoughts. What are thoughts and where do they come from? Thoughts are energy, consciousness. They are impulses of intelligence. I think thoughts are electrical energy and feelings are chemical. Every thought has a feeling. Good thoughts have good feelings and destructive thoughts have bad feelings and can cause disease. Thoughts come from the silent space between thoughts, this space or gap is where are creative insights arise as well as the Universal Mind (God) the gap is a space of higher consciousness.

There is another teacher of mindfulness meditation; Jon Kabat-Zinn, PhD gives an eight week course at the University of Massachusetts. His techniques are of value for those with cancer, heart disease and serious illness, pain and stress. He has written a book called "Full Catastrophe Living". I highly recommend this book. He also has tapes on Mindfulness Meditation.

The next three pages give a complete discussion including the exercise in Mindfulness Meditation by Deepak Chopra.

Although in the west today, meditation is thought in terms of stress management and relaxation, the true purpose is a spiritual one. The experience of your inner self is the most important; the body is the objective experience of our ideas, while the mind is the subjective experience of them.

The body and the mind are ever changing. The one who is having the experience is beyond time and space it is the real you – it is our soul. The real you is a non-local field of information that is trapped in space and time by the body and mind. Your soul, the thinker of thoughts, finds expression through the mind and body, but when the mind and brain are destroyed, nothing happens to the real you. The real you is in the silent space between thoughts. Our thoughts come from time gap between thoughts. The space between thoughts is where are cosmic consciousness is located. This silent space is where the Universal Mind (God, unconditional love, light, and nature) resides. The insights are in this space. This is a silence filled with infinite possibility of thoughts, a field of pure potentiality.

The practice of meditation takes our awareness from a disturbed state of consciousness in the mind and the world of physical objects to the undisturbed state of consciousness in the realm of the soul and spirit. Through regular practice we gain access to the infinite storehouse of knowledge—the ultimate reality of creation. Who are we really? We are pure unbounded consciousness. Our individual awareness and cosmic awareness are the same, as the microcosm goes, so does the macrocosm. Mindfulness Meditation is an excellent way to get started.

The mindfulness mediation technique is a simple meditation procedure that can create a deep state of relaxation in your mind and body. As the mind quiets down but remains awake you will experience deeper, more silent levels of awareness. (Deepak Chopra-Jour Ney into healing).

1. Start by sitting comfortably in a quiet place where you will have a minimum amount of disturbance.
2. Close your eyes.
3. Breathe normally and naturally and gently allow your awareness to be on your breathing. Simply observe your breath, trying not to control it or alter it in any conscious way.
4. As you observe your breath, you may notice that it changes of its own accord. It may vary in speed, rhythm or depth and there may even be occasions when your breath seems to stop for a time. Whatever happens with your breathing, innocently observe it without trying to cause or initiate any change. (Remember that when you are relaxed your breath changes from shallow, rapid and irregular to deep, slow and regular).
5. You will find that at times your attention drifts away from your breath and you are thinking about other things or listening to noises outside. Whenever you notice you are not observing your breath, gently bring your attention back to your breathing.
6. If, during the meditation, you notice that you are focusing on some feeling, mood or expectation, treat this as you would any other thought and gently bring your attention back to your breathing.
7. Practice this meditation technique for fifteen minutes.
8. At the end of the fifteen minutes, keep your eyes closed and just sit easily for two to three minutes. Allow yourself to come out of the meditation gradually before opening your eyes and resuming your activity.

It is recommended that you practice this mindfulness meditation technique for about fifteen minutes twice a day in the morning and evening, you can also use this technique during the day when you are upset. During the meditation you will have three experiences.

You may feel bored and your mind may become filled with thoughts is an indication that stresses and emotions are being released. By continuing the meditation you will remove these impurities from your mind and body. You may fall asleep. If you fall asleep this means you need more rest during the day. You may slip into the "gap" when the breath becomes very settled and refined; you slip into the gap between thoughts, beyond sound, beyond breath.

If you stay rested, take care of yourself and take time to commit to meditation. You are bound to get in touch with your inner self. You will tap into your cosmic mind, the silent spaces between your thoughts. This is your inner intelligence that mirrors the wisdom of the universe. Trust this inner wisdom and all your dreams will come true.

Herman Hess writes, "Within you there is a stillness and sanctuary to which you can retreat at any time and be yourself", this sanctuary is a simple awareness of comfort which can't be violated by the turmoil of events. This place feels no trauma and stores no hurt. It is the healing mental space that one seeks to find in meditation. A quiet mind is all you need. When life is full, it is only love and when awareness is full it brings only love. Every thought in our awareness starts its journey from the source of life as love and nothing else. The use of love is to heal, when it flows without effort from the depth of self, love creates health. I would like to share with you a poem that sums up perfectly for me the whole topic of disease and our part in it:

> Each moment of love,
> Each moment of giving,
> Each moment of joy,
> Is a moment of living.
>
> Each moment of anger,
> Each moment of lying,
> Each moment of fear
> Is a moment of dying.
>
> All our moments add together,
> Like the digits in a sum,
> And the answer tells us plainly,
> Whether life or death will come.

When there are times when life isn't working, I remind myself of the poem who am I?

I am somebody!

I am bright, capable and lovable.
I am teachable and learn easily.
I tell the truth and am a gentle listener
I respect myself and others.
I am cooperative and responsible for my feelings and choices.
I see the highest and best in myself and others and
support that with my thoughts, words and actions.
I use time wisely because it is valuable.
I am the best me I can be each day.
I am somebody!
I am love.

LEVEL SEVEN: THE NATURE OF SPIRIT

"We are spiritual beings with human experiences. There are spiritual solutions to all problems if we remain connected to God," Dr. Wayne Dwyer.

Who are you?

So far, we have given our attention to the physical, mental and emotional aspects of ourselves plus considerable time to relaxation techniques, now in the seventh level we will embrace the domain of the spirit. This domain is different and is vitally important in the journey through cancer. Most of us out of necessity live our lives on the surface of things. The best metaphor is the ocean and the waves. The surface of the waves represents the domain of daily living, our daily lives. The waves can be choppy and turbulent or placid, the waves can be very turbulent after a diagnosis of cancer, but the bottom of the ocean is always still and peaceful.

The journey through cancer is a time when it is vitally important to look beneath the surface into the vast depths that are untouchable by the most turbulent waves. The deepest level of our inner self, our higher consciousness, unbounded consciousness, the ocean of awareness is where you find your true self. The purpose of my life is to know and love my true self-the timeless eternal essence of God, of spirit, and of all beings and to be a powerful presence of love, joy, wisdom, compassion, awareness and truth for myself and others. The profound serenity that underlies our everyday experiences in essence is the real, real world. By discovering the realm of spirit, your understanding of reality will be expanded and your life will never be the same.

Cancer and its treatments may be so overwhelming that the possibility of another reality may seem inconceivable, but it does exist.

The window of reality opens up when you sit quietly and allow the mind to calm down and begin to look within your own self. There you will find a different world that can never be reached through thought, effort or activity of any kind, a gentle silent awareness and presence of love and joy that has been the heart of every being. By entering the dimension of being that is untouched in the physical, mental and emotional realms, the peaks and valleys of the cancer journey are softened.

A genuine sense of peace and serenity can appear in the midst of the fiercest storms – that is of tremendous benefit to everyone, the realm of spirit, includes not only love and joy but physical healing as well. Entering the realm of spirit – Finding our spiritual essence is an intimate process of self-discovery. Most often it takes place through time spent in silence, in meditation and prayer, in nature, and in communication with family, friends, and loved ones and other patients.

Drugs and radiation may kill cancer cells but they don't make a human being healthy or joyful. That power comes from the spirit. Spontaneous remissions do occur and they enter your body through your soul – yet even the soul is not the deepest truth of who you are. The ultimate source of who you are is "you are the ocean", not the wave, by recognizing your real identity as the ocean (pure potentiality, all possibilities) rather than the wave you can find freedom not only from cancer but even from birth and death.

For both classical Buddhism and Vedic tradition of India however, the experience of an isolated, independent self is an illusion.

Clinging to the false idea of an independent self is regarded as the fundamental cause of suffering, illness, disease and death that human beings experience over and over again. When the inside of our separateness is dispelled, the interconnectedness of everything is clearly seen and understood. We are all connected. We are connected to the one God, universal love and cosmic consciousness. When we are separated from the One, problems arise, so does illness, disease and even cancer. Buddha saw and understood the illusion of separate self. Albert Einstein arrived at the same conclusion: "A human being is part of the whole, called by us the universe, a part limited in time and space, he experiences himself, his thoughts and feelings as something separated from the rest . . . . a kind of optical delusion of consciousness."

We are not the mind, we are not the body, we are not the universe, but the mind, the body and the universe are within us.

What is the ultimate cause of cancer?

In the worldview, cancer is caused by Oncogenes or tumor suppressor gene derangements. These derangements are caused by various toxins in the external world or by events in the internal world, precipitated by hormones, biochemical changes or by inherited genetic predisposition. This is the cause of cancer at the relative level.

The ultimate cause might be God or the devil, or some random event without any meaning. Finally, there is what I consider the enlightened view. Nothing exists independently from our own perception, in truth; we are not separated from anything in the universe.

THE NATURE OF SPIRIT

Who we are is indeed the pure ocean of awareness out of which everything arises and falls away again. The ultimate serenity of spirit that the patients discover in Level Seven is linked with the experience of oneness with all of existence. An additional aspect of this involves the recognition of who we are at the deepest level is also never truly touched by the storms of existence. When there is a storm at sea, at the very bottom of the ocean there is stillness. No matter how turbulent the waves appear on the surface, the bottom of the ocean remains silent and untouched. For the cancer patient, the turbulent, choppy suface, the waves appear real, but in every moment, at the deepest level of reality, the timeless, dimensionless, inner self is untouched by it.

It is important to remember that I am in no way suggesting that we ignore the outer world, the domain of doing, which includes the sensory experience, everyday life, and comprehensive cancer treatment. But in Level Seven, there is another possibility. The possibility to embrace the domain of being that exists simultaneously with the domain of doing. The domain of being is the ultimate healing journey, (in being there is no ego no self, just non-doing as in mindfulness meditation.)

This being, non-doing, opens the door to our true nature, our true self. The truth of who we really are beyond time and space, beyond what can be seen and known. The truth of who we are is not separate in any way from God, the cosmos and all that exists,

How is this related to the cause of cancer?

As long as you regard yourself as an individual being that is isolated and separate from others and from creation itself, you will experience yourself subject to the laws of nature, physics and biology.

Support groups allow us to connect to others which aides healing. Each of us experiences the results of our own actions, both positive and negative, which is called Karma. Karma is the law of cause and effect whatever you sow, so shall you reap. The individual soul wants to grow and expand and express the fullness of itself. If you water and nourish a plant, it will grow. If you don't it will die. Getting cancer means that the seed of this experience has been planted by our own thoughts, feelings and actions at some point in the past. Since we are not separate from all that exists, there are no "events" that occur "out there" without our involvement but knowing why is not the most important thing to move forward in your journey. "Why me" is a disempowering question.

HOW DO I WANT TO BE REMEMBERED?
1-I LOVED MY WIFE
2-1 LOVED MY CHILDREN
3-I LOVED MYSELF, GOD AND OTHERS
4-I ENJOYED LEARNING AND TEACHING
5-I ENJOYED WRITING ABOUT HEALTH TO HELP OTHERS
6-I WANTED TO MAKE A DIFFERENCE. A POSITIVE CHANGE

1.

IMPOTENCE IS ON THE RISE

There are many reasons for the lack of potency. Marital discord, fear of failure to perform, personal problems and financial problems, to name a few.

What can we do to improve our sexual performance? One way is to see yourself as a teenager with an abundance of testosterone. As a teenager with an abundance of testosterone, it becomes easy to have a penile erection and again have the morning erection.

As we get older we lose the morning erection. We must change our thinking and regress to an earlier phase of life particularly a teenager.

We can enhance our potency by bio-identical hormone replacement of testosterone. This is done by using testosterone cream in the morning; place the cream on our inner thighs. In addition to the cream, use two and one half milligrams of Cialis on a daily basis. This combination, Cialis and testosterone causes an erection. We need to have an erection and maintain the erection for penetration. Imagine, see and feel yourself as a sexual powerhouse, believe it and achieve it.

Resource – Sue Johnson Sex Specialist

ANTI-AGING MEDICINE IS THE MEDICINE OF THE FUTURE

Anti-aging medicine does not treat symptoms or disease. Anti-aging medicine looks for the cause and prevention of illness. Conventional medicine treats disease.

I am not interested in treating disease, I want to find the cause and prevention of disease. Hormonal replacement therapy plays an important part in anti-aging medicine. Bio-identical replacement is a must. I replace my bio-identical testosterone cream in the morning, and my Progesterone cream in the evening. These creams are rubbed into my thighs.

The progesterone cream used in the evening, makes me sleepy and I fall asleep easily when I use this cream. I am a member of the AAMA-Anti-Aging Medicine Group and I attend their conferences. I have an anti-aging doctor who checks my blood and treats the cause. My anti-aging physician is Dr. James Cennamo DO. If there is an abnormality in my blood he corrects it.

WE ARE WHAT WE EAT AND WHAT WE DO

A healthy diet is made of fruits and veggies grains, beans and nuts. Cancer and anti-aging depends on a nutritious diet. We should juice with cruciferous vegetables and fruits. After juicing add a Superfood to the juice.

Greens plus 3 tablespoonfuls plus Aloe Vera 1 oz. and fruits and veggies. 90% of cancer patients depend on good nutrition. Refer to Charles Simeone in his book cancer nutrition.

In addition to a healthy diet we should do resistant exercises, yoga, Pilates, walking and riding a bicycle for 30 minutes. Brisk walking for 30 minutes on a daily basis.

INDEX

Index-Part II Breast Cancer